Cram101 Textbook Outlines to accompany:

Nursing Diagnosis : Application to Clinical Practice

Lynda Juall Carpenito-Moyet, 12th Edition

Learning System

Cram101 Textbook Outlines is a learning system. The notes in this book are the highlights of your textbook, you will never have to highlight a book again.

How to use this book. Take this book to class, it is your notebook for the lecture. The notes and highlights on the left hand side of the pages follow the outline and order of the textbook. All you have to do is follow along while your instructor presents the lecture. Circle the items emphasized in class and add other important information on the right side. With Cram101 Textbook Outlines you'll spend less time writing and more time listening. Learning becomes more efficient.

Cram101.com Online

Increase your studying efficiency by using Cram101.com's practice tests and online reference material. It is the perfect complement to Cram101 Textbook Outlines. Use self-teaching matching tests or simulate in-class testing with comprehensive multiple choice tests, or simply use Cram's true and false tests for quick review. Cram101.com even allows you to enter your in-class notes for an integrated studying format combining the textbook notes with your class notes.

Visit **www.Cram101.com**, click Sign Up at the top of the screen, and enter **DK73DW8114** in the promo code box on the registration screen. Your access to www.Cram101.com is discounted by 50% because you have purchased this book. Sign up and stop highlighting textbooks forever.

 ISBN(s): 9781618124579. PUBE-2.2011529

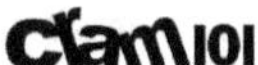

Nursing Diagnosis : Application to Clinical Practice
Lynda Juall Carpenito-Moyet, 12th

CONTENTS

Nursing diagnosis	A nursing diagnosis is part of the nursing process and is a clinical judgment about individual, family, or community experiences/responses to actual or potential health problems/life processes. Nursing diagnoses are developed based on data obtained during the nursing assessment. NANDA The primary organization for defining, dissemination and integration of standardized nursing diagnoses worldwide is NANDA-International formerly known as the North American Nursing Diagnosis Association.
Clinical practice	Good Clinical practice is an international quality standard that is provided by International Conference on Harmonisation (ICH), an international body that defines standards, which governments can transpose into regulations for clinical trials involving human subjects. Good Clinical practice guidelines include protection of human rights as a subject in clinical trial. It also provides assurance of the safety and efficacy of the newly developed compounds.
Diagnosis	Diagnosis is the identification of the nature of anything, either by process of elimination or other analytical methods. diagnosis is used in many different disciplines, with slightly different implementations on the application of logic and experience to determine the cause and effect relationships. Below are given as examples and tools used by the respective professions in medicine, science, engineering, business.
Nursing diagnoses	A nursing diagnosis is a standardized statement about the health of a client (who can be an individual, a family) for the purpose of providing nursing care. nursing diagnoses are developed based on data obtained during the nursing assessment. The main organization for defining standard diagnoses in North America is the North American Nursing Diagnosis Association, now known as NANDA-International.
Perfusion	In physiology, Perfusion is the process of nutritive delivery of arterial blood to a capillary bed in the biological tissue.`

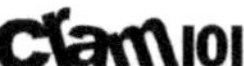

	Tests of adequate Perfusion are a part of patient triage performed by medical or emergency personnel in a mass casualty incident. Perfusion can be calculated with the following formula, where P_A is mean arterial pressure, P_V is mean venous pressure, and R is vascular resistance: 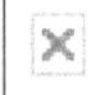 The term $P_A - P_V$ is sometimes presented as ΔP, for the change in pressure. The terms `Perfusion` and `Perfusion pressure` are sometimes used interchangeably, but the equation should make clear that resistance can have an effect on the Perfusion, but not on the Perfusion pressure.
Nurse	A Nurse is a healthcare professional who, in collaboration with other members of a health care team, is responsible for: treatment, safety, and recovery of acutely or chronically ill individuals; health promotion and maintenance within families, communities and populations; and, treatment of life-threatening emergencies in a wide range of health care settings. Nurses perform a wide range of clinical and non-clinical functions necessary to the delivery of health care, and may also be involved in medical and nursing research. Both Nursing roles and education were first defined by Florence Nightingale, following her experiences caring for the wounded in the Crimean War.
Nurse anesthetist	A nurse anesthetist is a nurse who specializes in the administration of anesthesia. In the United States, a Certified Registered Nurse Anesthetist is an advanced practice registered nurse (APRN) who has acquired graduate-level education and board certification in the specialty of anesthesia. The American Association of Nurse Anesthetists' (AANA) is the national association that represents more than 92% of nurse anesthetists in the United States.

Nursing practice	Nursing practice is the actual provision of nursing care. In providing care, nurses are implementing the nursing care plan which is based on the client`s initial assessment. This is based around a specific nursing theory which will be selected as appropriate for the care setting.
Cryptosporidiosis	Cryptosporidiosis, also known as crypto, is a parasitic disease caused by Cryptosporidium, a protozoan parasite in the phylum Apicomplexa. It affects the intestines of mammals and is typically an acute short-term infection. It is spread through the fecal-oral route, often through contaminated water; the main symptom is self-limiting diarrhea in people with intact immune systems.
Spiritual distress	Spiritual distress is a disturbance in a person`s belief system. As an approved nursing diagnosis, Spiritual distress is defined as `a disruption in the life principle that pervades a person`s entire being and that integrates and transcends one`s biological and psychological nature.` Authors in the field of nursing who contributed to the definition of the characteristics of Spiritual distress used indicators to validate diagnoses. The following manifestations of Spiritual distress are a part of an abstract data gathered by LearnWell Resources, Inc from the studies of Mary Elizabeth O`Brien and is used as a Spiritual Assessment Guide to present alterations in spiritual integrity.
NANDA	NANDA International (formerly the NANDA) is a professional organization of nurses standardized nursing terminology that was officially founded in 1982 and develops, researches, disseminates and refines the nomenclature, criteria, and taxonomy of nursing diagnoses. In 2002, NANDA relaunched as NANDA International in response to the broadening scope of its membership. NANDA International published Nursing Diagnosis quarterly, which became the International Journal of Nursing Terminologies and Classifications in 2002.Other related international associations are AENTDE, AFEDI and JSND History

In 1973 the First National Conference on the Classification of Nursing Diagnoses was held in St. Louis, Missouri which created the National Conference Group, a task force to standardize nursing terminology.

Nursing process

The nursing process is a process by which nurses deliver care to individuals, families, and/or communities and is supported by nursing theories. The nursing process was originally an adapted form of problem-solving and is classified as a deductive theory.

Phases of the nursing process

The nursing process is a client-centered, goal-oriented method of caring that provides a framework to nursing care.

Nursing diagnosis	A nursing diagnosis is part of the nursing process and is a clinical judgment about individual, family, or community experiences/responses to actual or potential health problems/life processes. Nursing diagnoses are developed based on data obtained during the nursing assessment. NANDA The primary organization for defining, dissemination and integration of standardized nursing diagnoses worldwide is NANDA-International formerly known as the North American Nursing Diagnosis Association.
Diagnosis	Diagnosis is the identification of the nature of anything, either by process of elimination or other analytical methods. diagnosis is used in many different disciplines, with slightly different implementations on the application of logic and experience to determine the cause and effect relationships. Below are given as examples and tools used by the respective professions in medicine, science, engineering, business.
Nursing diagnoses	A nursing diagnosis is a standardized statement about the health of a client (who can be an individual, a family) for the purpose of providing nursing care. nursing diagnoses are developed based on data obtained during the nursing assessment. The main organization for defining standard diagnoses in North America is the North American Nursing Diagnosis Association, now known as NANDA-International.
Herpes simplex	Herpes simplex is a viral disease caused by both herpes simplex virus 1 and herpes simplex virus 2 (HSV-2). Infection with the herpes virus is categorized into one of several distinct disorders based on the site of infection. Oral herpes, the visible symptoms of which are colloquially called cold sores, infects the face and mouth.
Herpes zoster	Herpes zoster commonly known as shingles and also known as zona, is a viral disease characterized by a painful skin rash with blisters in a limited area on one side of the body, often in a stripe. The initial infection with varicella zoster virus (VZV) causes the acute (short-lived) illness chickenpox, and generally occurs in children and young people. Once an episode of chickenpox has resolved, the virus is not eliminated from the body but can go on to cause shingles--an illness with very different symptoms--often many years after the initial infection.

Virus	A Virus is a small infectious agent that can only replicate inside the cells of another organism. Viruses are too small to be seen directly with a light microscope. Viruses infect all types of organisms, from animals and plants to bacteria and archaea.
Rubella	Rubella, commonly known as German measles, is a disease caused by the Rubella virus. The name `Rubella` is derived from the Latin, meaning little red. Rubella is also known as German measles because the disease was first described by German physicians in the mid-eighteenth century.
Measles	Measles is an infection of the respiratory system caused by a virus, specifically a paramyxovirus of the genus Morbillivirus. Morbilliviruses, like other paramyxoviruses, are enveloped, single-stranded, negative-sense RNA viruses. Symptoms include fever, cough, runny nose, red eyes and a generalized, maculopapular, erythematous rash.
Sympathetic	The word Sympathetic means different things in different contexts. · In neurology and neuroscience, the Sympathetic nervous system is a part of the autonomic nervous system. · In music theory, Sympathetic strings are strings on a musical instrument that resonate without contact. · In psychology, sympathy is a feeling of compassion or identification with another. · In religion, magic, and anthropology, sympathy is the belief that like affects like, that something can be influenced through its relationship with another thing.
Injury	Injury is damage or harm caused to the structure or function of the body caused by an outside agent or force, which may be physical or chemical, and either by accident or intentional. Personal Injury also refers to damage caused to the reputation of another rather than physical harm to the body. A severe and life-threatening Injury is referred to as a physical trauma. · Bruise is a hemorrhage under the skin caused by contusion. · Wound: cuts and grazes are injuries to or through the skin, that cause bleeding (i.e., a laceration). · Burns are injuries caused by excess heat, chemical exposure, or sometimes cold (frostbite). · Fractures are injuries to bones.

· Joint dislocation is a displacement of a bone from its normal joint, such as a dislocated shoulder or finger.

· Concussion is mild traumatic brain Injury caused by a blow, without any penetration into the skull or brain.

· Sprain is an Injury which occurs to ligaments caused by a sudden over stretching; a strain injures muscles.

· Shock is a serious medical condition where the tissues cannot obtain sufficient oxygen and nutrients.

· Amputation is the removal of a body extremity by trauma or surgery.

· Serious bodily Injury is any Injury or injuries to the body that substantially risks death of the victim.

Nervous system

The nervous system is a network of specialized cells that coordinate the actions of an animal and send signals from one part of its body to another. These cells send signals either as electrochemical waves traveling along thin fibers called axons, or as chemicals released onto other cells. The nervous system is composed of neurons and other specialized cells called glial cells .

Spinal cord

The spinal cord is a long, thin, tubular bundle of nervous tissue and support cells that extends from the brain. The brain and spinal cord together make up the central nervous system. The spinal cord extends down to the space in between the first and second lumbar vertebrae.

Syndrome

In medicine and psychology, the term syndrome refers to the association of several clinically recognizable features, signs (observed by a physician), symptoms (reported by the patient), phenomena or characteristics that often occur together, so that the presence of one feature alerts the physician to the presence of the others. In recent decades the term has been used outside of medicine to refer to a combination of phenomena seen in association.

The term syndrome derives from its Greek roots and means literally `run together`, as the features do.

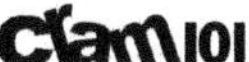

Clinical practice	Good Clinical practice is an international quality standard that is provided by International Conference on Harmonisation (ICH), an international body that defines standards, which governments can transpose into regulations for clinical trials involving human subjects. Good Clinical practice guidelines include protection of human rights as a subject in clinical trial. It also provides assurance of the safety and efficacy of the newly developed compounds.
Constipation	Constipation refers to bowel movements that are infrequent and/or hard to pass. Constipation is a common cause of painful defecation. Severe constipation includes obstipation (failure to pass stools or gas) and fecal impaction .
Mechanical ventilation	In medicine, mechanical ventilation is a method to mechanically assist or replace spontaneous breathing. This may involve a machine called a ventilator or the breathing may be assisted by a physician or other suitable person compressing a bag or set of bellows. Traditionally divided into negative-pressure ventilation, where air is essentially sucked into the lungs, or positive pressure ventilation, where air (or another gas mix) is pushed into the trachea.
Physical therapy	Physical therapy is a health care profession that provides treatment to individuals to develop, maintain and restore maximum movement and function throughout life. This includes providing treatment in circumstances where movement and function are threatened by aging, injury, disease or environmental factors. Physical therapy is concerned with identifying and maximizing quality of life and movement potential within the spheres of promotion, prevention, treatment/intervention, habilitation and rehabilitation.
Interventions	Interventions is a book by Noam Chomsky, an American linguist, MIT professor, and political activist. Published in May 2007, Interventions is a collection of 44 op-ed articles, post-9/11, from September 2002, through March 2007. After 9/11, Noam Chomsky began writing short, roughly 1000 word concise articles, distributed by The New York Times Syndicate as op-eds. They were widely picked up overseas but rarely in the US and only in smaller regional or local papers.
Barriers	Barriers is a British children's television series made by Tyne Tees Television for ITV between 1981 and 1982.

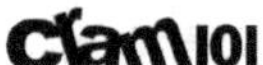

	The series starred Benedict Taylor as Billy Stanyon, a teenager facing up to the loss of his parents in a sailing accident only to discover that he was adopted. Billy then sets off on a journey to find his real parents that takes him across Europe.
Detection	In general, detection is the extraction of particular information from a larger stream of information without specific cooperation from or synchronization with the sender. In the history of radio communications, the term 'detector' was first used for a device that detected the simple presence or absence of a radio signal, since all communications were in Morse code. The term is still in use today to describe a component that extracts a particular signal from all of the electromagnetic waves present.

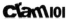

Chapter 3. PART III: Chapter 5 - Chapter 6

Diagnosis	Diagnosis is the identification of the nature of anything, either by process of elimination or other analytical methods. diagnosis is used in many different disciplines, with slightly different implementations on the application of logic and experience to determine the cause and effect relationships. Below are given as examples and tools used by the respective professions in medicine, science, engineering, business.
Nursing diagnoses	A nursing diagnosis is a standardized statement about the health of a client (who can be an individual, a family) for the purpose of providing nursing care. nursing diagnoses are developed based on data obtained during the nursing assessment. The main organization for defining standard diagnoses in North America is the North American Nursing Diagnosis Association, now known as NANDA-International.
Nursing diagnosis	A nursing diagnosis is part of the nursing process and is a clinical judgment about individual, family, or community experiences/responses to actual or potential health problems/life processes. Nursing diagnoses are developed based on data obtained during the nursing assessment. NANDA The primary organization for defining, dissemination and integration of standardized nursing diagnoses worldwide is NANDA-International formerly known as the North American Nursing Diagnosis Association.
Herpes simplex	Herpes simplex is a viral disease caused by both herpes simplex virus 1 and herpes simplex virus 2 (HSV-2). Infection with the herpes virus is categorized into one of several distinct disorders based on the site of infection. Oral herpes, the visible symptoms of which are colloquially called cold sores, infects the face and mouth.
Herpes zoster	Herpes zoster commonly known as shingles and also known as zona, is a viral disease characterized by a painful skin rash with blisters in a limited area on one side of the body, often in a stripe. The initial infection with varicella zoster virus (VZV) causes the acute (short-lived) illness chickenpox, and generally occurs in children and young people. Once an episode of chickenpox has resolved, the virus is not eliminated from the body but can go on to cause shingles--an illness with very different symptoms--often many years after the initial infection.

Virus

A Virus is a small infectious agent that can only replicate inside the cells of another organism. Viruses are too small to be seen directly with a light microscope. Viruses infect all types of organisms, from animals and plants to bacteria and archaea.

Interventions

Interventions is a book by Noam Chomsky, an American linguist, MIT professor, and political activist. Published in May 2007, Interventions is a collection of 44 op-ed articles, post-9/11, from September 2002, through March 2007. After 9/11, Noam Chomsky began writing short, roughly 1000 word concise articles, distributed by The New York Times Syndicate as op-eds. They were widely picked up overseas but rarely in the US and only in smaller regional or local papers.

Physical therapy

Physical therapy is a health care profession that provides treatment to individuals to develop, maintain and restore maximum movement and function throughout life. This includes providing treatment in circumstances where movement and function are threatened by aging, injury, disease or environmental factors.

Physical therapy is concerned with identifying and maximizing quality of life and movement potential within the spheres of promotion, prevention, treatment/intervention, habilitation and rehabilitation.

Interventions

Interventions is a book by Noam Chomsky, an American linguist, MIT professor, and political activist. Published in May 2007, Interventions is a collection of 44 op-ed articles, post-9/11, from September 2002, through March 2007. After 9/11, Noam Chomsky began writing short, roughly 1000 word concise articles, distributed by The New York Times Syndicate as op-eds. They were widely picked up overseas but rarely in the US and only in smaller regional or local papers.

Mucous membrane

The Mucous membranes are linings of mostly endodermal origin, covered in epithelium, which are involved in absorption and secretion. They line various body cavities that are exposed to the external environment and internal organs. It is at several places continuous with skin: at the nostrils, the lips, the ears, the genital area, and the anus.

Rubella

Rubella, commonly known as German measles, is a disease caused by the Rubella virus. The name `Rubella` is derived from the Latin, meaning little red. Rubella is also known as German measles because the disease was first described by German physicians in the mid-eighteenth century.

Measles

Measles is an infection of the respiratory system caused by a virus, specifically a paramyxovirus of the genus Morbillivirus. Morbilliviruses, like other paramyxoviruses, are enveloped, single-stranded, negative-sense RNA viruses. Symptoms include fever, cough, runny nose, red eyes and a generalized, maculopapular, erythematous rash.

Standardization	Standardization or standardisation is the process of developing and agreeing upon technical standards. A standard is a document that establishes uniform engineering or technical specifications, criteria, methods, processes, or practices. Some standards are mandatory while others are voluntary.
Risk factor	A risk factor is a variable associated with an increased risk of disease or infection. risk factors are correlational and not necessarily causal, because correlation does not imply causation. For example, being young cannot be said to cause measles, but young people are more at risk as they are less likely to have developed immunity during a previous epidemic.
Cardiovascular	The circulatory system is an organ system that passes nutrients (such as amino acids and electrolytes), gases, hormones, blood cells, etc. to and from cells in the body to help fight diseases and help stabilize body temperature and pH to maintain homeostasis. This system may be seen strictly as a blood distribution network, but some consider the circulatory system as composed of the cardiovascular system, which distributes blood, and the lymphatic system, which distributes lymph.
Respiratory	The respiratory system`s function is to allow gas exchange to all parts of the body. The space between the alveoli and the capillaries, the anatomy or structure of the exchange system, and the precise physiological uses of the exchanged gases vary depending on the organism. In humans and other mammals, for example, the anatomical features of the respiratory system include airways, lungs, and the respiratory muscles.
Respiratory system	The respiratory system`s function is to allow gas exchange to all parts of the body. The space between the alveoli and the capillaries, the anatomy or structure of the exchange system, and the precise physiological uses of the exchanged gases vary depending on the organism. In humans and other mammals, for example, the anatomical features of the respiratory system include airways, lungs, and the respiratory muscles.
Cardiac	The heart is a muscular organ found in all vertebrates that is responsible for pumping blood throughout the blood vessels by repeated, rhythmic contractions. The term cardiac means 'related to the heart' and comes from the Greek καρδιΐ¬, kardia, for 'heart.' The vertebrate heart is composed of cardiac muscle, which is an involuntary striated muscle tissue found only within this organ. The average human heart, beating at 72 beats per minute, will beat approximately 2.5 billion times during an average 66 year lifespan.

Chronic disease | In medicine, a chronic disease is a disease that is long-lasting or recurrent. The term chronic describes the course of the disease, or its rate of onset and development. A chronic course is distinguished from a recurrent course; recurrent diseases relapse repeatedly, with periods of remission in between.

Constipation | Constipation refers to bowel movements that are infrequent and/or hard to pass. Constipation is a common cause of painful defecation. Severe constipation includes obstipation (failure to pass stools or gas) and fecal impaction .

Fatigue | Fatigue atigue (also called exhaustion, lethargy, languidness, languor, lassitude, and listlessness) is a state of awareness. It can describe a range of afflictions, varying from a general state of lethargy to a specific work-induced burning sensation within one`s muscles. It can be both physical and mental.

Bed rest | Bed rest is a medical treatment involving a period of consistent (day and night) recumbence in bed. It is used as a treatment for an illness or medical condition, especially when prescribed or chosen rather than resulting from severe prostration or imminent death. Even though most patients in hospitals spend most of their time in the hospital beds, Bed rest more often refers to an extended period of recumbence at home.

Concept | There are two prevailing theories in contemporary philosophy which attempt to explain the nature of concepts. The representational theory of mind proposes that concepts are mental representations, while the semantic theory of concepts holds that they are abstract objects. Ideas are taken to be concepts, although abstract concepts do not necessarily appear to the mind as images as some ideas do.

Sleep | Sleep is a naturally recurring state of relatively suspended sensory and motor activity, characterized by total or partial unconsciousness and the inactivity of nearly all voluntary muscles. It is distinguished from quiet wakefulness by a decreased ability to react to stimuli, and it is more easily reversible than hibernation or coma. It is observed in all mammals, all birds, and many reptiles, amphibians, and fish.

COPD | Chronic obstructive pulmonary disease (COPD) refers to chronic bronchitis and emphysema, a pair of two commonly co-existing diseases of the lungs in which the airways become narrowed. This leads to a limitation of the flow of air to and from the lungs causing shortness of breath. In contrast to asthma, the limitation of airflow is poorly reversible and usually gets progressively worse over time.

Anxiety | Anxiety is a psychological and physiological state characterized by cognitive, somatic, emotional, and behavioral components. These components combine to create an unpleasant feeling that is typically associated with uneasiness, fear, or worry.

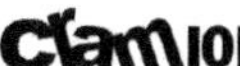

	Anxiety is a generalized mood condition that occurs without an identifiable triggering stimulus. As such, it is distinguished from fear, which occurs in the presence of an observed threat. Additionally, fear is related to the specific behaviors of escape and avoidance, whereas anxiety is the result of threats that are perceived to be uncontrollable or unavoidable.
Panic	Panic is a sudden fear which dominates or replaces thinking and often affects groups of people or animals. panics typically occur in disaster situations, or violent situations (such as robbery, home invasion, a shooting rampage, etc). which may endanger the overall health of the affected group.
Cryptosporidiosis	Cryptosporidiosis, also known as crypto, is a parasitic disease caused by Cryptosporidium, a protozoan parasite in the phylum Apicomplexa. It affects the intestines of mammals and is typically an acute short-term infection. It is spread through the fecal-oral route, often through contaminated water; the main symptom is self-limiting diarrhea in people with intact immune systems.
Dyspnea	Dyspnea or dyspnoea , from Latin dyspnoea, from Greek dyspnoia from dyspnoos, shortness of breath), also called shortness of breath or air hunger, is a debilitating symptom that is the experience of unpleasant or uncomfortable respiratory sensations. It is a common symptom of numerous medical disorders, particularly those involving the cardiovascular and respiratory systems; Dyspnea on exertion is the most common presenting complaint for people with respiratory impairment. Dyspnea has been more specifically defined by the American Thoracic Society as the 'subjective experience of breathing discomfort that consists of qualitatively distinct sensations that vary in intensity.
Paralysis	Paralysis is the complete loss of muscle function for one or more muscle groups. Paralysis can cause loss of feeling or loss of mobility in the affected area. Paralysis is most often caused by damage in the nervous system, especially the spinal cord.

Alcoholism	Alcoholism has multiple and sometimes conflicting definitions. In common and historic usage, Alcoholism is any condition that results in the continued consumption of alcoholic beverages, despite health problems and negative social consequences. Modern medical definitions describe Alcoholism as a disease and addiction which results in a persistent use of alcohol despite negative consequences. In the 19th and early 20th centuries, alcoholism, also referred to as dipsomania described a preoccupation with, or compulsion toward the consumption of, alcohol and/or an impaired ability to recognize the negative effects of excessive alcohol consumption.
Immunodeficiency	Immunodeficiency is a state in which the immune system`s ability to fight infectious disease is compromised or entirely absent. Most cases of Immunodeficiency are acquired (`secondary`) but some people are born with defects in the immune system, or primary Immunodeficiency. Transplant patients take medications to suppress their immune system as an anti-rejection measure, as do some patients suffering from an over-active immune system.
Syndrome	In medicine and psychology, the term syndrome refers to the association of several clinically recognizable features, signs (observed by a physician), symptoms (reported by the patient), phenomena or characteristics that often occur together, so that the presence of one feature alerts the physician to the presence of the others. In recent decades the term has been used outside of medicine to refer to a combination of phenomena seen in association. The term syndrome derives from its Greek roots and means literally `run together`, as the features do.
Hyperventilation	In medicine, Hyperventilation is the state of breathing faster and/or deeper than necessary, bringing about lightheadedness and other undesirable symptoms often associated with panic attacks. Hyperventilation can also be a response to metabolic acidosis, a condition that causes acidic blood pH levels. Counterintuitively, such side effects are not precipitated by the sufferer`s lack of oxygen or air.
Body temperature	Normal human Body temperature, also known as normothermia or euthermia, is a concept that depends upon the place in the body at which the measurement is made, and the time of day and level of activity of the body. Although the value 37.0 °C (98.6 °F) is the commonly accepted average core Body temperature, the value of 36.8±0.7 °C, or 98.2±1.3 °F is an average oral (under the tongue) measurement. Rectal measurements, or measurements taken directly inside the body cavity, are typically slightly higher.

Convection	Convection is the movement of molecules within fluids (i.e. liquids, gases and rheids). It cannot take place in solids, since neither bulk current flows or significant diffusion can take place in solids. Convection is one of the major modes of heat transfer and mass transfer.
Fever	Fever is a frequent medical sign that describes an increase in internal body temperature to levels above normal. fever is most accurately characterized as a temporary elevation in the body`s thermoregulatory set-point, usually by about 1-2 °C . fever is caused by an elevation in the thermoregulatory set-point, causing typical body temperature (generally and problematically considered to be 37 °C or 98.6 °F) to rise, and effector mechanisms are enacted as a result.
Hyperthermia	Hyperthermia is an elevated body temperature due to failed thermoregulation. Hyperthermia occurs when the body produces or absorbs more heat than it can dissipate. When the elevated body temperatures are sufficiently high, Hyperthermia is a medical emergency and requires immediate treatment to prevent disability and death.
Hypothermia	Hypothermia is a condition in which an organism`s temperature drops below that required for normal metabolism and body functions. In warm-blooded animals, core body temperature is maintained near a constant level through biologic homeostasis or thermoregulation. However, when the body is exposed to cold, its internal mechanisms may be unable to replenish the heat that is being lost to the organism`s surroundings.
Radiation	In physics, radiation describes any process in which energy emitted by one body travels through a medium or through space, ultimately to be absorbed by another body. Non-physicists often associate the word with ionizing radiation (e.g., as occurring in nuclear weapons, nuclear reactors, and radioactive substances), but it can also refer to electromagnetic radiation (i.e., radio waves, infrared light, visible light, ultraviolet light, and X-rays) which can also be ionizing radiation, to acoustic radiation, or to other more obscure processes. What makes it radiation is that the energy radiates (i.e., it travels outward in straight lines in all directions) from the source.
Physiology	Physiology is the science of the functioning of living systems. It is a subcategory of biology. In physiology, the scientific method is applied to determine how organisms, organ systems, organs, cells and biomolecules carry out the chemical or physical function that they have in a living system.

Chapter 3. PART III: Chapter 5 - Chapter 6

Sepsis	Sepsis is a serious medical condition that is characterized by a whole-body inflammatory state (called a systemic inflammatory response syndrome or SIRS) and the presence of a known or suspected infection. The body may develop this inflammatory response to microbes in the blood, urine, lungs, skin, or other tissues. An incorrect layman`s term f is blood poisoning, more aptly applied to Septicemia, below.
Pulmonary embolism	Pulmonary embolism is a blockage of the main artery of the lung or one of its branches by a substance that has travelled from elsewhere in the body through the bloodstream (embolism). Usually this is due to embolism of a thrombus (blood clot) from the deep veins in the legs, a process termed venous thromboembolism. A small proportion is due to the embolization of air, fat or amniotic fluid.
Thermoregulation	Thermoregulation is the ability of an organism to keep its body temperature within certain boundaries, even when the surrounding temperature is very different. This process is one aspect of homeostasis: a dynamic state of stability between an animal`s internal environment and its external environment (the study of such processes in zoology has been called ecophysiology or physiological ecology). If the body is unable to maintain a normal temperature and it increases significantly above normal, a condition known as hyperthermia occurs.
Hypothalamus	The hypothalamus is a portion of the brain that contains a number of small nuclei with a variety of functions. One of the most important functions of the hypothalamus is to link the nervous system to the endocrine system via the pituitary gland (hypophysis). The hypothalamus is located below the thalamus, just above the brain stem.
Glucose	Glucose, a monosaccharide (or simple sugar) also known as grape sugar, blood sugar, is a very important carbohydrate in biology. The living cell uses it as a source of energy and metabolic intermediate. glucose is one of the main products of photosynthesis and starts cellular respiration in both prokaryotes (bacteria and archaea) and eukaryotes (animals, plants, fungi, and protists).
Hyperglycemia	Hyperglycemia, hyperglycaemia, or high blood sugar is a condition in which an excessive amount of glucose circulates in the blood plasma. This is generally a blood glucose level of 10+ mmol/L (180 mg/dl), but symptoms may not start to become noticeable until later numbers such as 15-20+ mmol/L (270-360 mg/dl)or 15.2-32.6 mmol/L. However, chronic levels exceeding 125 mg/dl can produce organ damage.

	The origin of the term is Greek: hyper-, meaning excessive; -glyc-, meaning sweet; and -emia, meaning \`of the blood\`.
Hypoglycemia	Hypoglycemia or hypoglycæmia is the medical term for a state produced by a lower than normal level of blood glucose. The term literally means \`under-sweet blood\` . hypoglycemia can produce a variety of symptoms and effects but the principal problems arise from an inadequate supply of glucose as fuel to the brain, resulting in impairment of function .
Fecal incontinence	Fecal incontinence is the loss of regular control of the bowels. Involuntary excretion and leaking are common occurrences for those affected. Subjects relating to defecation are often socially unacceptable, thus those affected may be beset by feelings of shame and humiliation.
Spinal cord	The spinal cord is a long, thin, tubular bundle of nervous tissue and support cells that extends from the brain. The brain and spinal cord together make up the central nervous system. The spinal cord extends down to the space in between the first and second lumbar vertebrae.
Injury	Injury is damage or harm caused to the structure or function of the body caused by an outside agent or force, which may be physical or chemical, and either by accident or intentional. Personal Injury also refers to damage caused to the reputation of another rather than physical harm to the body. A severe and life-threatening Injury is referred to as a physical trauma. · Bruise is a hemorrhage under the skin caused by contusion. · Wound: cuts and grazes are injuries to or through the skin, that cause bleeding (i.e., a laceration). · Burns are injuries caused by excess heat, chemical exposure, or sometimes cold (frostbite). · Fractures are injuries to bones. · Joint dislocation is a displacement of a bone from its normal joint, such as a dislocated shoulder or finger. · Concussion is mild traumatic brain Injury caused by a blow, without any penetration into the skull or brain. · Sprain is an Injury which occurs to ligaments caused by a sudden over stretching; a strain injures muscles.

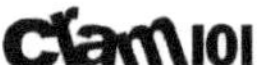

· Shock is a serious medical condition where the tissues cannot obtain sufficient oxygen and nutrients.

· Amputation is the removal of a body extremity by trauma or surgery.

· Serious bodily Injury is any Injury or injuries to the body that substantially risks death of the victim.

Perfusion

In physiology, Perfusion is the process of nutritive delivery of arterial blood to a capillary bed in the biological tissue.`

Tests of adequate Perfusion are a part of patient triage performed by medical or emergency personnel in a mass casualty incident.

Perfusion can be calculated with the following formula, where P_A is mean arterial pressure, P_V is mean venous pressure, and R is vascular resistance:

The term $P_A - P_V$ is sometimes presented as ΔP, for the change in pressure.

The terms `Perfusion` and `Perfusion pressure` are sometimes used interchangeably, but the equation should make clear that resistance can have an effect on the Perfusion, but not on the Perfusion pressure.

Postpartum

Postnatal is the period beginning immediately after the birth of a child and extending for about six weeks. Another term would be Postpartum period, as it refers to the mother . Less frequently used is puerperium.

Mastitis

Mastitis is the inflammation of breast tissue. S. aureus is the most common etiological organism responsible, but S. epidermidis and streptococci are occasionally isolated as well.

Popular usage of the term mastitis varies by geographic region.

Nipple

In its most general form, a Nipple is a structure from which a fluid emanates. More specifically, it is the projection on the breasts of a mammal by which breast milk is delivered to a mother`s young.

In the anatomy of mammals, a Nipple or mammary papilla or teat is a small projection of skin containing the outlets for 15-20 lactiferous ducts arranged cylindrically around the tip.

Body image

Body image is a term which may refer to a person's perception of his or her own physical appearance, or the interpretation of the body by the brain. Essentially, Body image describes how one perceives one's appearance to be in relation to others, which in many cases may be dramatically different from one's objective physical condition or how one is actually perceived by others.

A 2007 report by the American Psychological Association found that a culture-wide sexualization of girls (and women) was contributing to increased female anxiety associated with Body image.

Arrhythmia

Cardiac Arrhythmia is a term for any of a large and heterogeneous group of conditions in which there is abnormal electrical activity in the heart. The heart beat may be too fast or too slow, and may be regular or irregular.

Some Arrhythmias are life-threatening medical emergencies that can result in cardiac arrest and sudden death. Others cause symptoms such as an abnormal awareness of heart beat (palpitations), and may be merely annoying. Still others may not be associated with any symptoms at all, but predispose toward potentially life-threatening stroke or embolus.

Bradycardia

Bradycardia , as applied to adult medicine, is defined as a resting heart rate of under 60 beats per minute, though it is seldom symptomatic until the rate drops below 50 beat/min. It may cause 'heart attacks' in some patients or cardiac arrest. This occurs because someone with bradycardia may not be pumping enough oxygen to their own heart causing heart attack-like symptoms.

Cardiac output

Cardiac output is the volume of blood being pumped by the heart, in particular by a ventricle in a minute. This is measured in dm^3/min (1 dm^3 equals 1000 cm^3 or 1 litre). An average Cardiac output would be 5 L/min for a human male and 4.5 L/min for a female.

Chapter 3. PART III: Chapter 5 - Chapter 6

Spinal shock	Spinal shock was first defined by Whytt in 1750 as a loss of sensation accompanied by motor paralysis with initial loss but gradual recovery of reflexes, following a spinal cord injury (SCI) -- most often a complete transection. Reflexes in the spinal cord caudal to the SCI are depressed (hyporeflexia) or absent (areflexia), while those rostral to the SCI remain unaffected. Note that the `shock` in Spinal shock does not refer to circulatory collapse.
Vascular	In zoology and medicine, `vascular` means `related to blood vessels`, which are part of the Circulatory system. An organ or tissue that is vascularized is heavily endowed with blood vessels and thus richly supplied with blood. In botany, plants with a dedicated transport system for water and nutrients are called vascular plants.
Nursing home	A nursing home, convalescent home, Skilled Nursing Unit (SNU), care home or rest home provides a type of care of residents: it is a place of residence for people who require constant nursing care and have significant deficiencies with activities of daily living. Residents include the elderly and younger adults with physical or mental disabilities. Eligible adults 18 or older can stay in a skilled nursing facility to receive physical, occupational, and other rehabilitative therapies following an accident or illness.
Malaise	Malaise is a feeling of general discomfort or uneasiness, an `out of sorts` feeling, often the first indication of an infection or other disease. Malaise is often defined in medicinal research as a `general feeling of being unwell`. The term is also often used figuratively in other contexts; for example, `economic Malaise` refers to an economy that is stagnant or in recession.
Insomnia	Insomnia is a symptom of any of several sleep disorders, characterized by persistent difficulty falling asleep or staying asleep despite the opportunity. insomnia is a symptom, not a stand-alone diagnosis or a disease. By definition, insomnia is `difficulty initiating or maintaining sleep, or both` and it may be due to inadequate quality or quantity of sleep.
Back pain	Back pain is pain felt in the back that usually originates from the muscles, nerves, bones, joints or other structures in the spine. The pain can often be divided into neck pain, upper Back pain, lower Back pain or tailbone pain. It may have a sudden onset or can be a chronic pain; it can be constant or intermittent, stay in one place or radiate to other areas.

Ischemia	In medicine, Ischemia is a restriction in blood supply, generally due to factors in the blood vessels, with resultant damage or dysfunction of tissue. It may also be spelled ischaemia or ischæmia.Also means local anemia in a given part of a body sometimes resulting from vasoconstriction, thrombosis or embolism. Rather than hypoxia (a more general term denoting a shortage of oxygen, usually a result of lack of oxygen in the air being breathed), Ischemia is an absolute or relative shortage of the blood supply to an organ, i.e. a shortage of oxygen, glucose and other blood-borne fuels.
Addiction	An addiction is an obsession, compulsion, or excessive psychological dependence, such as: drug addiction problem gambling, ergomania, compulsive overeating, shopping addiction, computer addiction, video game addiction, pornography addiction, television addiction, etc. In medicine, an addiction is a chronic neurobiological disorder that has genetic, psychosocial, and environmental dimensions and is characterized by one of the following: the continued use of a substance despite its detrimental effects, impaired control over the use of a drug (compulsive behavior), and preoccupation with a drug's use for non-therapeutic purposes (i.e. craving the drug). addiction is often accompanied by the presence of deviant behaviors (for instance stealing money and forging prescriptions) that are used to obtain a drug.
Withdrawal	Withdrawal can refer to any sort of separation, but is most commonly used to describe the group of symptoms that occurs upon the abrupt discontinuation/separation or a decrease in dosage of the intake of medications, recreational drugs, and/or alcohol. In order to experience the symptoms of Withdrawal, one must have first developed a physical dependence (often referred to as chemical dependency). This happens after consuming one or more of these substances for a certain period of time, which is both dose dependent and varies based upon the drug consumed.
Abuse	Abuse is defined as: Abuse of information typically involves a breach of confidence or plagiarism. Abuse of power, in the form of 'malfeasance in office' or 'official misconduct', is the commission of an unlawful act, done in an official capacity, which affects the performance of official duties. Malfeasance in office is often grounds for a for cause removal of an elected official by statute or recall election.

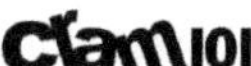

Drug addiction	Drug addiction is a pathological or abnormal condition which arises due to frequent drug use. The disorder of addiction involves the progression of acute drug use to the development of drug-seeking behavior, the vulnerability to relapse, and the decreased, slowed ability to respond to naturally rewarding stimuli. The Diagnostic and Statistical Manual of Mental Disorders, Fourth Edition (DSM-IV) has categorized three stages of addiction: preoccupation/anticipation, binge/intoxication, and withdrawal/negative affect.
Pharmacokinetics	Pharmacokinetics is a branch of pharmacology dedicated to the determination of the fate of substances administered externally to a living organism. In practice, this discipline is applied mainly to drug substances, though in principle it concerns itself with all manner of compounds ingested or otherwise delivered externally to an organism, such as nutrients, metabolites, hormones, toxins, etc. pharmacokinetics is often studied in conjunction with pharmacodynamics.
Chronic pain	Chronic pain has several different meanings in medicine. Traditionally, the distinction between acute and chronic pain has relied upon an arbitrary interval of time from onset; the two most commonly used markers being 3 months and 6 months since the initiation of pain, though some theorists and researchers have placed the transition from acute to chronic pain at 12 months. Others apply acute to pain that lasts less than 30 days, chronic to pain of more than six months duration, and subacute to pain that lasts from one to six months.
Opioid	An opioid is a chemical that works by binding to opioid receptors, which are found principally in the central nervous system and the gastrointestinal tract. The receptors in these two organ systems mediate both the beneficial effects and the side effects of opioids. The analgesic effects of opioids are due to decreased perception of pain, decreased reaction to pain as well as increased pain tolerance.
Nausea	Nausea, is the sensation of unease and discomfort in the upper stomach and head with an urge to vomit. An attack of Nausea is known as a qualm. Nausea which affects the stomach is sometimes called wamble.
Sedation	Sedation is a medical procedure involving the administration of sedative drugs, generally to facilitate a medical procedure with local anaesthesia.

	sedation is now typically used in procedures such as endoscopy, vasectomy,RSI (Rapid Sequence Intubation), or minor surgery and in dentistry for reconstructive surgery, some cosmetic surgeries, removal of wisdom teeth, or for high-anxiety patients. sedation methods in dentistry include inhalation sedation oral sedation, and intravenous (IV) sedation.
Opioid	An opioid is a chemical that works by binding to opioid receptors, which are found principally in the central nervous system and the gastrointestinal tract. The receptors in these two organ systems mediate both the beneficial effects and the side effects of opioids. The analgesic effects of opioids are due to decreased perception of pain, decreased reaction to pain as well as increased pain tolerance.
Analgesic	An analgesic is any member of the group of drugs used to relieve pain (achieve analgesia). Analgesic drugs act in various ways on the peripheral and central nervous systems; they include paracetamol (para-acetylaminophenol, also known in the US as acetaminophen), the non-steroidal anti-inflammatory drugs (NSAIDs) such as the salicylates, and opioid drugs such as morphine and opium. They are distinct from anesthetics, which reversibly eliminate sensation.
Latex allergy	Latex allergy is a medical term encompassing a range of allergic reactions to natural rubber latex. Latex is known to cause 2 of the 4 (or 5) types of hypersensitivity. The most serious and rare form, type I is an immediate and potentially life-threatening reaction, not unlike the severe reaction some people have to bee stings.
Stimulation	Stimulation is the action of various agents (stimuli) on muscles, nerves, or a sensory end organ, by which activity is evoked; especially, the nervous impulse produced by various agents on nerves, or a sensory end organ, by which the part connected with the nerve is thrown into a state of activity.

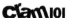

The word is also often used metaphorically. For example, an interesting or fun activity can be described as "stimulating", regardless of its physical effects on nerves.

Barriers

Barriers is a British children's television series made by Tyne Tees Television for ITV between 1981 and 1982.

The series starred Benedict Taylor as Billy Stanyon, a teenager facing up to the loss of his parents in a sailing accident only to discover that he was adopted. Billy then sets off on a journey to find his real parents that takes him across Europe.

Receptive aphasia

Receptive aphasia, also known as Wernicke`s aphasia, fluent aphasia, is a type of aphasia often (but not always) caused by neurological damage to Wernicke`s area in the brain (Brodmann area 22, in the posterior part of the superior temporal gyrus of the dominant hemisphere). This is not to be confused with Wernicke`s encephalopathy or Wernicke-Korsakoff syndrome. The aphasia was first described by Carl Wernicke and its understanding substantially advanced by Norman Geschwind.

Aphasia

Aphasia is an acquired language disorder in which there is an impairment of any language modality. This may include difficulty in producing or comprehending spoken or written language. Traditionally, 'Aphasia' suggests the total impairment of language ability, and 'Dysphasia' a degree of impairment less than total.

Touch

The somatosensory system is a diverse sensory system comprising the receptors and processing centres to produce the sensory modalities such as touch, temperature, proprioception (body position), and nociception (pain). The sensory receptors cover the skin and epithelia, skeletal muscles, bones and joints, internal organs, and the cardiovascular system. While touch is considered one of the five traditional senses, the impression of touch is formed from several modalities; In medicine, the colloquial term touch is usually replaced with somatic senses to better reflect the variety of mechanisms involved.

Geriatrics

Geriatrics is the branch of medicine that focuses on health care of the elderly. It aims to promote health and to prevent and treat diseases and disabilities in older adults.

	geriatrics was separated from internal medicine as a distinct entity in the same way that pediatrics is separated from adult internal medicine and neonatology is separated from pediatrics.
Malnutrition	Malnutrition is the insufficient, excessive or imbalanced consumption of nutrients. A number of different nutrition disorders may arise, depending on which nutrients are under or overabundant in the diet. The World Health Organization cites Malnutrition as the gravest single threat to the world`s public health.
Telecommunication	Telecommunication is the transmission of signals over a distance for the purpose of communication. In earlier times, this may have involved the use of smoke signals, drums, semaphore, flags or heliograph. In modern times, Telecommunication typically involves the use of electronic devices such as telephones, television, radio or computers.
Comprehension	Comprehension has the following meanings: · In general usage, and more specifically in reference to education and psychology, it has roughly the same meaning as understanding. · Reading Comprehension measures the understanding of a passage of text · In logic, the Comprehension of an object is the totality of intensions, that is, properties or qualities, that it possesses. · Related to this, in Anglicanism, Comprehension refers to the theological inclusiveness and liturgical breadth thought to be integral to the definition of the tradition · In set theory, Comprehension is another name for the axiom schema of specification (or more specifically, the axiom schema of unrestricted specification). · A related term in computer science, list Comprehension, denotes an adaptation of mathematical set notation to represent infinite lists. Comprehensions are most closely associated with Haskell, but are available in other languages such as Python, Scheme and Common Lisp.

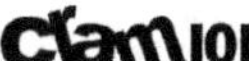

Chapter 3. PART III: Chapter 5 - Chapter 6

Electrolyte	In chemistry, an Electrolyte is any substance containing free ions that make the substance electrically conductive. The most typical Electrolyte is an ionic solution, but molten Electrolytes and solid Electrolytes are also possible. Electrolytes commonly exist as solutions of acids, bases or salts.
Electrolyte imbalances	Electrolytes play a vital role in maintaining homeostasis within the body. They help to regulate myocardial and neurological function, fluid balance, oxygen delivery, acid-base balance and much more. Electrolyte imbalances can develop by the following mechanisms: excessive ingestion; diminished elimination of an electrolyte; diminished ingestion or excessive elimination of an electrolyte.
Metabolism	Metabolism is the set of chemical reactions that happen in living organisms to maintain life. These processes allow organisms to grow and reproduce, maintain their structures, and respond to their environments. metabolism is usually divided into two categories.
Stroke	A stroke is the rapidly developing loss of brain function(s) due to disturbance in the blood supply to the brain. This can be due to ischemia (lack of glucose ' oxygen supply) caused by thrombosis or embolism or due to a hemorrhage. As a result, the affected area of the brain is unable to function, leading to inability to move one or more limbs on one side of the body, inability to understand or The traditional definition of stroke, devised by the World Health Organization in the 1970s, is a `neurological deficit of cerebrovascular cause that persists beyond 24 hours or is interrupted by death within 24 hours`.
Depression	Depression is a state of low mood and aversion to activity that can affect a person's thoughts, behaviour, feelings and physical well-being. It may include feelings of sadness, anxiety, emptiness, hopelessness, worthlessness, guilt, irritability, or restlessness. Depressed people may lose interest in activities that once were pleasurable, experience difficulty concentrating, remembering details, or making decisions, and may contemplate or attempt suicide.
Self-esteem	Self-esteem is a term used in psychology to reflect a person`s overall evaluation or appraisal of his or her own worth.  Self-esteem encompasses beliefs (for example, `I am competent-incompetent`) and emotions (for example, triumph-despair, pride-shame). Behavior may reflect Self-esteem.

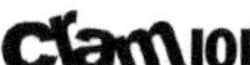

Catheter	In medicine, a catheter is a tube that can be inserted into a body cavity, duct, or vessel. catheters thereby allow drainage, injection of fluids, or access by surgical instruments. The process of inserting a catheter is catheterization.
Intravenous	Intravenous therapy or IV therapy is the giving of liquid substances directly into a vein. The word Intravenous simply means `within a vein`. Therapies administered Intravenously are often called specialty pharmaceuticals.
Intravenous therapy	Intravenous therapy or IV therapy is the giving of liquid substances directly into a [[vein]. The word intravenous simply means `within a vein`. Therapies administered intravenously are often called specialty pharmaceuticals.
Bladder	In anatomy, the urinary bladder is the organ that collects urine excreted by the kidneys prior to disposal by urination. A hollow muscular, and distensible (or elastic) organ, the bladder sits on the pelvic floor. Urine enters the bladder via the ureters and exits via the urethra.
Music therapy	Music therapy is an interpersonal process in which a trained music therapist uses music and all of its facets--physical, emotional, mental, social, aesthetic, and spiritual--to help clients to improve or maintain their health. Music therapists primarily help clients improve their observable level of functioning and self-reported quality of life in various domains (e.g., cognitive functioning, motor skills, emotional and affective development, behavior and social skills) by using music experiences (e.g., singing, songwriting, listening to and discussing music, moving to music) to achieve measurable treatment goals and objectives. Referrals to Music therapy services may be made by a treating physician or an interdisciplinary team consisting of clinicians such as physicians, psychologists, social workers, physical therapists, and occupational therapists.
Recreation	Recreation or fun is the expenditure of time in a manner designed for therapeutic refreshment of one`s body or mind. While leisure is more likely a form of entertainment or sleep, Recreation is active for the participant but in a refreshing and diverting manner. As people in the world`s wealthier regions lead increasingly sedentary lifestyles, the need for Recreation has increased.
Reminiscence therapy	Reminiscence therapy is used to counsel and support older people, and is an intervention technique with brain-injured patients. This form of therapeutic intervention respects the life and experiences of the individual with the aim to help the patient maintain good mental health.

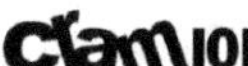

Often utilised in residential and nursing care settings, reminiscence therapy is also to be found in none-acute hospitals in the United Kingdom for example, especially those specialising in medical care for the elderly. In one approach, participants are guided by a trained person to reflect on a variety of aspects relating to their lives. This may be themed and centre on one period in time or it may be wider and reflect a guided discussion through an issue. The therapist may use music, photographs, replica documents, drama and sensory gardens to stimulate debate and discussion for the participants.

Pediatric

Pediatrics is the branch of medicine that deals with the medical care of infants, children, and adolescents. The upper age limit of such patients ranges from age 12 to 21, depending on the country. A medical practitioner who specializes in this area is known as a pediatrician.

Peristalsis

Peristalsis is a radially symmetrical contraction of muscles which propagates in a wave down the muscular tube. In humans, Peristalsis is found in the contraction of smooth muscles to propel contents through the digestive tract. Earthworms use a similar mechanism to drive their locomotion.

Encopresis

Encopresis, from the Greek κοπρος is involuntary 'fecal soiling' in children who have usually already been toilet trained. Children with encopresis often leak stool into their underwear.

The estimated prevalence of encopresis in 4-year-olds is ~1-3%.

Enema

An Enema is the procedure of introducing liquids into the rectum and colon via the anus. The increasing volume of the liquid causes rapid expansion of the lower intestinal tract, often resulting in very uncomfortable bloating, cramping, powerful peristalsis, a feeling of extreme urgency and complete evacuation of the lower intestinal tract.

Enemas can be carried out as treatment for medical conditions, such as constipation and encopresis, and as part of some alternative health therapies.

Laxative

Laxatives (also known as purgatives or aperients) are foods, compounds, or drugs taken to induce bowel movements or to loosen the stool, most often taken to treat constipation. Certain stimulant, lubricant, and saline laxatives are used to evacuate the colon for rectal and bowel examinations, and may be supplemented by enemas in that circumstance. Sufficiently high doses of laxatives will cause diarrhea.

Functional constipation	Functional constipation is constipation that does not have a physical (anatomical) or physiological (hormonal or other body chemistry) cause. It may have a neurological, psychological or psychosomatic cause. A person with Functional constipation may be healthy, yet has difficulty defecating.
Fecal impaction	A Fecal impaction is a solid, immobile bulk of human feces that can develop in the rectum as a result of chronic constipation.
Rectal examination	A rectal examination or rectal exam is an internal examination of the rectum such as by a physician or other healthcare professional. The digital rectal examination is a relatively simple procedure. The patient undresses, then is placed in a position where the anus is accessible (lying on the side, squatting on the examination table, bent over the examination table, or lying down with feet in stirrups).
Impaction	Impaction is a medical term used to describe several different types of blockage. Impaction is a pathological condition in humans when an impassable mass of stone-like faecal matter collects in the rectum. It frequently occurs as a result of dehydration, inactivity, and medications, such as narcotics or psychotropicagents, which slow the peristalsis, and increase the time that the colonic mucosa will extract moisture from the faecal bolus.
Biologic	Biologics include a wide range of medicinal products such as vaccines, blood and blood components, allergenics, somatic cells, gene therapy, tissues, and recombinant therapeutic proteins created by biological processes (as distinguished from chemistry). Biologics can be composed of sugars, proteins, or nucleic acids or complex combinations of these substances, or may be living entities such as cells and tissues. Biologics are isolated from a variety of natural sources -- human, animal, or microorganism -- and may be produced by biotechnology methods and other technologies.
Microorganism	A microorganism or microbe is an organism that is microscopic . The study of microorganisms is called microbiology, a subject that began with Anton van Leeuwenhoek`s discovery of microorganisms in 1675, using a microscope of his own design.

	microorganisms are very diverse; they include bacteria, fungi, archaea, and protists; microscopic plants (called green algae); and animals such as plankton and the planarian.
Pertussis	Pertussis, also known as whooping cough, is a highly contagious disease caused by the bacterium Bordetella pertussis. It is known to last for a duration of approximately 6 weeks before subsiding. The disease derives its name from the `whoop` sound made from the inspiration of air after a cough.
Viruses	A virus is a small infectious agent that can only replicate inside the cells of another organism. viruses are too small to be seen directly with a light microscope. viruses infect all types of organisms, from animals and plants to bacteria and archaea.
Ebola	Ebola is the virus Ebolavirus (EBOV), a viral genus, and the disease Ebola hemorrhagic fever (EHF), a viral hemorrhagic fever (VHF). The virus is named after the Ebola River Valley in the Democratic Republic of the Congo (formerly Zaire), which is near the site of the first recognized outbreak, a mission hospital run by Flemish nuns, in 1976. There are four recognised species within the Ebolavirus genus, which have a number specific strains. The Zaire virus is the type species, which is also the first discovered and the most lethal.
Erythema	Erythema is redness of the skin, caused by congestion of the capillaries in the lower layers of the skin. It occurs with any skin injury, infection, or inflammation. Erythema disappears on finger pressure (blanching), while purpura or bleeding in the skin and pigmentation do not.
Erythema infectiosum	Erythema infectiosum or fifth disease is one of several possible manifestations of infection by erythrovirus previously called parvovirus B19. The disease is also referred to as slapped cheek syndrome, slapcheek, slap face or slapped face. In Japan the disease is called `apple sickness` or `ringo-byou` , identified as a distinct condition in 1896 by T. Escherich, and given the name `Erythema infectiosum` in 1899.
Ricin	Ricin is a protein that is extracted from the castor bean (Ricinus communis). It can be either a white powder or a liquid in crystalline form. Ricin may cause allergic reactions, and is toxic, though the severity depends on the route of exposure.

Smallpox	Smallpox is an infectious disease unique to humans, caused by either of two virus variants, Variola major and Variola minor. The disease is also known by the Latin names Variola or Variola vera, which is a derivative of the Latin varius, meaning spotted, or varus, meaning `pimple`. The term `Smallpox` was first used in Europe in the 15th century to distinguish variola from the `great pox` .
Biological agent	A biological agent is a bacterium, virus, prion, fungus, or biological toxin that can be used in bioterrorism or biological warfare. More than 1200 different kinds of biological agents have been described and studied to date. Applying a slightly broader definition, some eukaryotes (for example parasites) and their associated toxins can be considered as biological agents.
Hemorrhagic fevers	The viral Hemorrhagic fevers are a diverse group of animal and human illnesses that are caused by five distinct families of RNA viruses: the Arenaviridae, Filoviridae, Bunyaviridae, Togaviridae, and Flaviviridae. All types of VHF are characterized by fever and bleeding disorders and all can progress to high fever, shock and death in extreme cases. Some of the VHF agents cause relatively mild illnesses, such as the Scandinavian nephropathia epidemica, while others, such as the African Ebola virus, can cause severe, life-threatening disease. · The Arenaviridae include the viruses responsible for Lassa fever and Argentine, Bolivian, Brazilian and Venezuelan Hemorrhagic fevers. · The Bunyaviridae include the members of the Hantavirus genus that cause hemorrhagic fever with renal syndrome (HFRS), the Crimean-Congo hemorrhagic fever (CCHF) virus from the Nairovirus genus, and the Rift Valley fever (RVF) virus from the Phlebovirus genus. · The Filoviridae include Ebola and Marburg viruses. · Finally, the Flaviviridae include dengue, yellow fever, and two viruses in the tick-borne encephalitis group that cause VHF: Omsk hemorrhagic fever virus and Kyasanur Forest disease virus.
German measles	Rubella, commonly known as German measles, is a disease caused by the rubella virus. The name `rubella` is derived from the Latin, meaning little red. Rubella is also known as German measles because the disease was first described by German physicians in the mid-eighteenth century.

Giardiasis	Giardiasis in humans is caused by the infection of the small intestine by a single-celled organism called Giardia lamblia. Giardiasis occurs worldwide with a prevalence of 20-30% in developing countries. Additionally, Giardia has a wide range of human and other mammalian hosts, thus making it very difficult to eliminate.
Hepatitis	Hepatitis implies inflammation of the liver characterized by the presence of inflammatory cells in the tissue of the organ. The name is from ancient Greek hepar , the root being hepat- (á¼¡πατ-), meaning liver, and suffix -itis, meaning \`inflammation\` (c. 1727). The condition can be self-limiting, healing on its own, or can progress to scarring of the liver.
Hepatitis A	Hepatitis A is an acute infectious disease of the liver caused by the Hepatitis A virus (HAV), which is most commonly transmitted by the fecal-oral route via contaminated food or drinking water. Every year, approximately 10 million people worldwide are infected with the virus. The time between infection and the appearance of the symptoms, (the incubation period), is between two and six weeks and the average incubation period is 28 days.
Environmental factors	In epidemiology, environmental factors are those determinants of disease that are not transmitted genetically or by infection. Apart from the true monogenic genetic disorders, environmental diseases may determine the development of disease in those genetically predisposed to a particular condition. Stress, physical and mental abuse, diet, exposure to toxins, pathogens, radiation and chemicals found in almost all personal care products and household cleaners are possible causes of a large segment of non-hereditary disease.
Statistics	Statistics is the science of making effective use of numerical data relating to groups of individuals or experiments. It deals with all aspects of this, including not only the collection, analysis and interpretation of such data, but also the planning of the collection of data, in terms of the design of surveys and experiments. A statistician is someone who is particularly versed in the ways of thinking necessary for the successful application of statistical analysis.
Stressor	In chemistry, a Stressor is something that either speeds up a reaction rate or keeps the reaction rate the same. Stressors include light, temperature and elevated sound levels. Stressors also include the phenomena of substance concentration (does not shift equilibrium), catalysis, substance surface area (speeds up the reaction rate), and the nature of the reactants.

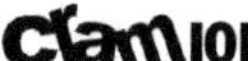

Chapter 3. PART III: Chapter 5 - Chapter 6

Child abuse	Child abuse is the physical or psychological/emotional mistreatment of children. In the United States, the Centers for Disease Control and Prevention (CDC) define child maltreatment as any act or series of acts of commission or omission by a parent or other caregiver that results in harm, potential for harm, or threat of harm to a child. Most child abuse occurs in a child's home, with a smaller amount occurring in the organizations, schools or communities the child interacts with.
Breast Cancer	Breast Cancer is a cancer that starts in the breast, usually in the inner lining of the milk ducts or lobules. There are different types of breast Cancer, with different stages (spread), aggressiveness, and genetic makeup. Survival varies greatly depending on those factors; with best treatment, 10-year disease-free survival varies from 98% to 10%.
Cancer	Cancer (medical term: malignant neoplasm) is a class of diseases in which a group of cells display uncontrolled growth (division beyond the normal limits), invasion (intrusion on and destruction of adjacent tissues), and). These three malignant properties of cancers differentiate them from benign tumors, which are self-limited, and do not invade or metastasize. Most cancers form a tumor but some, like leukemia, do not.
Coping strategies	The German Freudian psychoanalyst Karen Horney defined four so-called Coping strategies to define interpersonal relations, one describing psychologically healthy individuals, the others describing neurotic states. These are the strategies in which psychologically healthy people develop relationships. It involves compromise.
Barbiturates	Barbiturates are drugs that act as central nervous system depressants, and, by virtue of this, they produce a wide spectrum of effects, from mild sedation to total anesthesia. They are also effective as anxiolytics, hypnotics and as anticonvulsants. They have addiction potential, both physical and psychological.
Cannabis	Cannabis, also known as marijuana, marihuana, and ganja , among many other names, refers to any number of preparations of the Cannabis plant intended for use as a psychoactive drug. The most common form of Cannabis used as a drug is the dried herbal form. The typical herbal form of Cannabis consists of the flowers and subtending leaves and stalks of mature pistillate or female plants.

Chapter 3. PART III: Chapter 5 - Chapter 6

Cocaine

Cocaine is a crystalline tropane alkaloid that is obtained from the leaves of the coca plant. The name comes from 'coca' in addition to the alkaloid suffix -ine, forming Cocaine. It is a stimulant of the central nervous system and an appetite suppressant.

Hallucinogens

The general group of pharmacological agents commonly known as Hallucinogens can be divided into three broad categories: psychedelics, dissociatives, and deliriants. These classes of psychoactive drugs have in common that they can cause subjective changes in perception, thought, emotion and consciousness. Unlike other psychoactive drugs, such as stimulants and opioids, the Hallucinogens do not merely amplify familiar states of mind, but rather induce experiences that are qualitatively different from those of ordinary consciousness.

Abstinence

Abstinence is a voluntary restraint from indulging in bodily activities that are widely experienced as giving pleasure. Most frequently, the term refers to abstention from sexual intercourse, alcohol or food. The practice can arise from religious prohibitions or practical considerations.

Humanism

Humanism is a perspective common to a wide range of ethical stances that attaches importance to human dignity, concerns, and capabilities, particularly rationality. Although the word has many senses, its meaning comes into focus when contrasted to the supernatural or to appeals to authority. Since the nineteenth century, Humanism has been associated with an anti-clericalism inherited from the eighteenth-century Enlightenment philosophes.

Terminal illness

Terminal illness is a medical term popularized in the 20th century to describe an active and malignant disease that cannot be cured or adequately treated and that is reasonably expected to result in the death of the patient. This term is more commonly used for progressive diseases such as cancer or advanced heart disease than for trauma. In popular use, it indicates a disease which will end the life of the sufferer.

Diarrhea

In medicine, diarrhea , also spelled diarrhoea , is the condition of having frequent loose or liquid bowel movements. Acute diarrhea is a common cause of death in developing countries and the second most common cause of infant deaths worldwide. The loss of fluids through diarrhea can cause severe dehydration which is one cause of death in diarrhea sufferers.

Pressure ulcer

Pressure ulcers are lesions caused by many factors such as: unrelieved pressure; friction; humidity; shearing forces; temperature; age; continence and medication; to any part of the body, especially portions over bony or cartilaginous areas such as sacrum, elbows, knees, ankles etc. Although easily prevented and completely treatable if found early, bedsores are often fatal - even under the auspices of medical care - and are one of the leading iatrogenic causes of death reported in developed countries, second only to adverse drug reactions. Prior to the 1950s, treatment was ineffective until Doreen Norton showed that the primary cure and treatment was to remove the pressure by turning the patient every two hours.

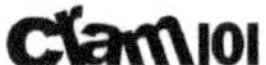

Venous blood	In the circulatory system, Venous blood is blood returning to the heart (in veins). With one exception (the pulmonary vein) this blood is deoxygenated and high in carbon dioxide, having released oxygen and absorbed CO_2 in the tissues. It is also typically warmer than arterial blood, has a lower pH, has lower concentrations of glucose and other nutrients, and has higher concentrations of urea and other waste products.
Blood flow	Blood flow is the flow of blood in the cardiovascular system. It can be calculated by dividing the vascular resistance into the pressure gradient. Mathematically, Blood flow is described by Darcy's law (which can be viewed as the fluid equivalent of Ohm's law) and approximately by Hagen-Poiseuille equation.
Contracture	A contracture, in a muscle or muscle fiber, usually refers to a continuous contraction in the absence of a stimulus, such as an action potential. A muscle contracture is a shortening of a muscle or joint.. It is usually in response to prolonged hypertonic spasticity in a concentrated muscle area, such as is seen in the tightest muscles of people with conditions like spastic cerebral palsy.
Retention	Retention can have the following meanings: · retention basin, instance retaining (e.g. water in the ground) · In learning: it is the ability to retain facts and figures in memory (spaced repetition) · Grade retention, in schools, keeping a student in the same grade for another year (that is, not promoting the student to the next higher grade with his/her classmates) · retention period, in Usenet, the time a news server holds a newsgroup posting before deleting it as no longer relevant · Judicial retention, in the United States court system, a process whereby a judge is periodically subject to a vote in order to remain in the position of judge · Urinary retention, the lack or inability to urinate

	· Employee retention, the ability to keep employees within an organization · retention agent is a process chemical `
Hypertension	Hypertension is a chronic medical condition in which the blood pressure is elevated. It is also referred to as high blood pressure or shortened to HT, HTN or HPN. The word `hypertension`, by itself, normally refers to systemic, arterial hypertension. hypertension can be classified as either essential (primary) or secondary.
Energy field disturbance	Energy field disturbance is a nursing diagnosis listed by NANDA (North American Nursing Diagnosis Association) that is rooted in energy medicine and alternative medicine. According to NANDA, energy field disturbance is defined as the disruption of the flow of energy, or aura, surrounding a person's being that results in a disharmony of the body, mind, and/or spirit. Defining characteristics • Perception of changes in movement • Perception of changes in sounds (tone or words) • Perception of temperature change (warmth or coolness) • Perception of visual changes (image or color) Nursing intervention According to NANDA, the recommended way to respond to energy disturbances is to explain the benefits of practices such as therapeutic touch and then to administer this care to the client.
Therapeutic touch	Therapeutic touch also called Non-Contact Therapeutic touch or Distance Healing, is an energy therapy claimed to promote healing and reduce pain and anxiety. Practitioners of Therapeutic touch claim that by placing their hands on, or near, a patient, they are able to detect and manipulate the patient`s putative energy field. Although there are currently (September 2009) 259 articles concerning Therapeutic touch on PubMed the quality of controlled research and tests is variable.

Radiation therapy	Radiation therapy (in North America)) , and , is the medical use of ionizing radiation as part of cancer treatment to control malignant cells (not to be confused with radiology, the use of radiation in medical imaging and diagnosis). Radiotherapy may be used for curative or adjuvant cancer treatment. It is used as palliative treatment (where cure is not possible and the aim is for local disease control or symptomatic relief) or as therapeutic treatment (where the therapy has survival benefit and it can be curative).
Rheumatoid arthritis	Rheumatoid arthritis is a chronic, systemic inflammatory disorder that may affect many tissues and organs, but principally attacks the joints producing an inflammatory synovitis that often progresses to destruction of the articular cartilage and ankylosis of the joints. rheumatoid arthritis can also produce diffuse inflammation in the lungs, pericardium, pleura, and sclera, and also nodular lesions, most common in subcutaneous tissue under the skin. Although the cause of rheumatoid arthritis is unknown, autoimmunity plays a pivotal role in its chronicity and progression.
Phobia	A phobia is an intense and persistent fear of certain situations, activities, things, animals, or people. The main symptom of this disorder is the excessive and unreasonable desire to avoid the feared subject. When the fear is beyond one`s control, and if the fear is interfering with daily life, then a diagnosis under one of the anxiety disorders can be made.
Threat	A Threat is an act of coercion wherein an act is proposed to elicit a negative response. It is a crime in many jurisdictions Brazilian jurisprudence does not treat as a crime a Threat that was proferred in a heated discussion.
Lymphoma	Lymphoma is a cancer that begins in the lymphocytes of the immune system and presents as a solid tumor of lymphoid cells. These malignant cells often originate in lymph nodes, presenting as an enlargement of the node (a tumor). lymphomas are closely related to lymphoid leukemias, which also originate in lymphocytes but typically involve only circulating blood and the bone marrow and do not usually form static tumours.
Urine	Urine is a liquid product of the body that is secreted by the kidneys by a process called urination and excreted through the urethra. Cellular metabolism generates numerous waste compounds, many rich in nitrogen, that require elimination from the bloodstream. This waste is eventually expelled from the body in a process known as micturition, the primary method for excreting water-soluble chemicals from the body.
Fluid balance	Fluid balance is the concept of human homeostasis that the amount of fluid lost from the body is equal to the amount of fluid taken in. Euvolemia is the state of normal body fluid volume.

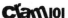

	Water is necessary for all life on Earth.
Specific gravity	Specific gravity, in the context of clinical pathology, is a urinalysis parameter commonly used in the evaluation of kidney function and can aid in the diagnosis of various renal diseases. The role of the kidneys in humans and other mammals is to aid in the clearance of various water-soluble molecules, including toxins, toxicants, and metabolic waste. The body excretes some of these waste molecules via urination, and the role of the kidney is to concentrate the urine, such that waste molecules can be excreted with minimal loss of water and nutrients.
Dehydration	Dehydration (hypohydration) is defined as excessive loss of body water. It is literally the removal of water from an object. In physiological terms, it entails a relative deficiency of water molecules in relation to other dissolved solutes.
Edema	Edema or oedema , formerly known as dropsy or hydropsy, is an abnormal accumulation of fluid beneath the skin or in one or more cavities of the body. Generally, the amount of interstitial fluid is determined by the balance of fluid homeostasis, and increased secretion of fluid into the interstitium or impaired removal of this fluid may cause edema. Five factors can contribute to the formation of edema: · It may be facilitated by increased hydrostatic pressure or, · reduced oncotic pressure within blood vessels; · by increased blood vessel wall permeability as in inflammation; · by obstruction of fluid clearance via the lymphatic; or, · by changes in the water retaining properties of the tissues themselves. Raised hydrostatic pressure often reflects retention of water and sodium by the kidney.
Lymphadenopathy	Lymphadenopathy is a term meaning `disease of the lymph nodes.` It is, however, almost synonymously used with `swollen/enlarged lymph nodes`. It could be due to infection, auto-immune disease, or malignancy.

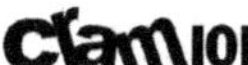

Inflammation of a lymph node is called lymphadenitis.

Bandage

A bandage is a piece of material used either to support a medical device such as a dressing or splint, or on its own to provide support to the body. Bandages are available in a wide range of types, from generic cloth strips, to specialised shaped bandages designed for a specific limb or part of the body, although bandages can often be improvised as the situation demands, using clothing, blankets or other material.

In common speech, the word "bandage" is often used to mean a dressing, which is used directly on a wound, whereas a bandage is technically only used to support a dressing, and not directly on a wound.

Pathophysiology

Pathophysiology is the study of the changes of normal mechanical, physical, and biochemical functions, either caused by a disease, or resulting from an abnormal syndrome. More formally, it is the branch of medicine which deals with any disturbances of body functions, caused by disease or prodromal symptoms.

An alternate definition is `the study of the biological and physical manifestations of disease as they correlate with the underlying abnormalities and physiological disturbances.`

The study of pathology and the study of Pathophysiology often involves substantial overlap in diseases and processes, but pathology emphasizes direct observations, while Pathophysiology emphasizes quantifiable measurements.

Mourning

Mourning is, in the simplest sense, synonymous with grief over the death of someone. The word is also used to describe a cultural complex of behaviours in which the bereaved participate or are expected to participate. Customs vary between different cultures and evolve over time, though many core behaviors remain constant.

Fetus

A Fetus is a developing mammal or other viviparous vertebrate after the embryonic stage and before birth. The plural is Fetuses.

In humans, the fetal stage of prenatal development starts at the beginning of the 11th week in gestational age, which is the 9th week after fertilization.

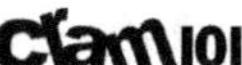

Chapter 3. PART III: Chapter 5 - Chapter 6

Autonomy	Autonomy is a concept found in moral, political, and bioethical philosophy. Within these contexts, it refers to the capacity of a rational individual to make an informed, un-coerced decision. In moral and political philosophy, Autonomy is often used as the basis for determining moral respectibility for one's actions.
Tuberculosis	Tuberculosis or TB (short for Tubercle Bacillus) is a common and often deadly infectious disease caused by mycobacteria, usually Mycobacterium tuberculosis in humans. tuberculosis usually attacks the lungs but can also affect other parts of the body. It is spread through the air, when people who have the disease cough, sneeze, or spit.
Motivational interviewing	Motivational interviewing refers to a counseling approach in part developed by clinical psychologists Professor William R Miller, Ph.D. and Professor Stephen Rollnick, Ph.D. It is a client-centered, semi-directive method of engaging intrinsic motivation to change behavior by developing discrepancy and exploring and resolving ambivalence within the client. Motivational interviewing recognizes and accepts the fact that clients who need to make changes in their lives approach counseling at different levels of readiness to change their behavior. If the counseling is mandated, they may never have thought of changing the behavior in question.
Health promotion	Health promotion has been defined by the World Health Organization`s 2005 Bangkok Charter f in a Globalized World as `the process of enabling people to increase control over their health and its determinants, and thereby improve their health`. The primary means of health promotion occur through developing healthy public policy that addresses the prerequisities of health such as income, housing, food security, employment, and quality working conditions. There is a tendency among public health officials and governments -- and this is especially the case in liberal nations such as Canada and the USA -- to reduce health promotion to health education and social marketing focused on changing behavioral risk factors.
Tobacco	Tobacco is an agricultural product processed from the leaves of plants in the genus Nicotiana. It can be consumed, used as an organic pesticide, and, in the form of nicotine tartrate, it is used in some medicines. In consumption it most commonly appears in the forms of smoking, chewing, snuffing, or dipping tobacco, or snus.
Adverse effect	In medicine, an adverse effect is a harmful and undesired effect resulting from a medication or other intervention such as surgery. An adverse effect may be termed a "side effect", when judged to be secondary to a main or therapeutic effect. If it results from an unsuitable or incorrect dosage or procedure, this is called a medical error and not a complication.

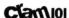

Primary prevention

Preventive medicine or preventive care refers to measures taken to prevent diseases, (or injuries) rather than curing them. It can be contrasted not only with curative medicine, but also with public health methods (which work at the level of population health rather than individual health). This takes place at primary, secondary and tertiary prevention levels.

· Primary prevention avoids the development of a disease.

Tertiary prevention

Preventive medicine or preventive care refers to measures taken to prevent diseases, (or injuries) rather than curing them or treating their symptoms. The term contrasts in method with curative and palliative medicine, and in scope with public health methods (which work at the level of population health rather than individual health).

This takes place at primary, secondary and Tertiary prevention levels.

· Primary prevention avoids the development of a disease.

Body mass index

The body mass index or Quetelet index, is a statistical measurement which compares a person's weight and height. Though it does not actually measure the percentage of body fat, it is used to estimate a healthy body weight based on how tall a person is. Due to its ease of measurement and calculation, it is the most widely used diagnostic tool to identify weight problems within a population, usually whether individuals are underweight, overweight or obese.

Nicotine

Nicotine is an alkaloid found in the nightshade family of plants (Solanaceae) which constitutes approximately 0.6-3.0% of dry weight of tobacco, with biosynthesis taking place in the roots, and accumulating in the leaves. It functions as an antiherbivore chemical with particular specificity to insects; therefore Nicotine was widely used as an insecticide in the past, and currently Nicotine analogs such as imidacloprid continue to be widely used.

In low concentrations , the substance acts as a stimulant in mammals and is the main factor responsible for the dependence-forming properties of tobacco smoking.

Weight	In the physical sciences, the weight of an object is the magnitude, W, of the force that must be applied to an object in order to support it (i.e. hold it at rest) in a gravitational field. The weight of an object in static equilibrium equals the magnitude of the gravitational force acting on the object, less the effect of its buoyancy in any fluid in which it might be immersed. Near the surface of the Earth, the acceleration due to gravity is approximately constant; this means that an object`s weight near the surface of the Earth is roughly proportional to its mass.
Meningitis	Meningitis is inflammation of the protective membranes covering the brain and spinal cord, known collectively as the meninges. The inflammation may be caused by infection with viruses, bacteria, or other microorganisms, and less commonly by certain drugs. Meningitis can be life-threatening because of the inflammation`s proximity to the brain and spinal cord; therefore the condition is classified as a medical emergency.
Menopause	Menopause is the permanent cessation of reproductive fertility occurring some time before the end of the natural lifespan. The term was originally coined to describe this reproductive change in human females, where the end of fertility is traditionally indicated by the permanent stopping of monthly menstruation or `menses`. The word `Menopause` literally means the `end of monthly cycles` from the Greek words pausis and the word root men from mensis meaning (month).
Osteoporosis	Osteoporosis is a disease of bone that leads to an increased risk of fracture. In osteoporosis the bone mineral density (BMD) is reduced, bone microarchitecture is disrupted, and the amount and variety of proteins in bone is altered. osteoporosis is defined by the World Health Organization (WHO) in women as a bone mineral density 2.5 standard deviations below peak bone mass (20-year-old healthy female average) as measured by DXA; the term `established osteoporosis` includes the presence of a fragility fracture.
Passive smoking	Passive smoking is the inhalation of smoke, called secondhand smoke (SHS) or environmental tobacco smoke (ETS), from tobacco products used by others. It occurs when tobacco smoke permeates any environment, causing its inhalation by people within that environment. Scientific evidence shows that exposure to secondhand tobacco smoke causes disease, disability, and death.
Influenza	Influenza, commonly referred to as the flu, is an infectious disease caused by RNA viruses of the family Orthomyxoviridae (the Influenza viruses), that affects birds and mammals. The name Influenza is Italian and means `influence` . The most common symptoms of the disease are chills, fever, sore throat, muscle pains, severe headache, coughing, weakness and general discomfort.

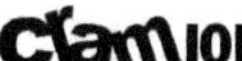

Pneumonia	Pneumonia is an abnormal inflammatory condition of the lung. It is often characterized as including inflammation of the parenchyma of the lung (that is, the alveoli) and abnormal alveolar filling with fluid (consolidation and exudation). The alveoli are microscopic air-filled sacs in the lungs responsible for absorbing oxygen.
Cytomegalovirus	Cytomegalovirus is a herpes viral genus of the Herpesviruses group: in humans it is commonly known as HCMV or Human Herpesvirus 5 . CMV belongs to the Betaherpesvirinae subfamily of Herpesviridae, which also includes Roseolovirus. Other herpesviruses fall into the subfamilies of Alphaherpesvirinae (including HSV 1 and 2 and varicella) or Gammaherpesvirinae (including Epstein-Barr virus).
Perioperative	The perioperative period, less commonly spelled the peroperative period, is the time period describing the duration of a patient's surgical procedure; this commonly includes ward admission, anesthesia, surgery, and recovery. Perioperative generally refers to the three phases of surgery: preoperative, intraoperative, and postoperative. The goal of perioperative care is to provide better conditions for patients before operation, during operation, and after operation.
Neglect	Neglect is a passive form of abuse in which the perpetrator is responsible to provide care for a victim who is unable to care for oneself, but fails to provide adequate care to meet the victim`s needs, thereby resulting in the victim`s demise. Neglect may include failing to provide sufficient supervision, nourishment, medical care or other needs for which the victim is helpless to provide for him/her/itself. The victim may be a child, physically or mentally disabled adult, animal, plant, or inanimate object.
Spiritual distress	Spiritual distress is a disturbance in a person`s belief system. As an approved nursing diagnosis, Spiritual distress is defined as `a disruption in the life principle that pervades a person`s entire being and that integrates and transcends one`s biological and psychological nature.` Authors in the field of nursing who contributed to the definition of the characteristics of Spiritual distress used indicators to validate diagnoses.

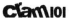

	The following manifestations of Spiritual distress are a part of an abstract data gathered by LearnWell Resources, Inc from the studies of Mary Elizabeth O`Brien and is used as a Spiritual Assessment Guide to present alterations in spiritual integrity.
Skin	The skin is the outer covering of the body. In humans, it is the largest organ of the integumentary system made up of multiple layers of mesodermal tissue, and guards the underlying muscles, bones, ligaments and internal organs. skin of a different nature exists in amphibians, reptiles, birds.
Damage	Damage is the physical stress, wear and tear, or breakage of something but may also more specifically refer to:
Motor system	The Motor system is the part of the central nervous system that is involved with movement. It consists of the pyramidal and extrapyramidal system. The motor pathway also called pyramidal tract or the corticospinal tract start in the motor center of the cerebral cortex.
Nervous system	The nervous system is a network of specialized cells that coordinate the actions of an animal and send signals from one part of its body to another. These cells send signals either as electrochemical waves traveling along thin fibers called axons, or as chemicals released onto other cells. The nervous system is composed of neurons and other specialized cells called glial cells .
Central	A central or intermediate group of three or four large glands is imbedded in the adipose tissue near the base of the axilla. Its afferents are the efferent vessels of all the preceding groups of axillary glands; its efferents pass to the subclavicular group.
Mycosis	Mycosis is a condition in which fungi pass the resistance barriers of the human or animal body and establish infections. Mycoses are classified according to the tissue levels initially colonized: Superficial mycoses - limited to the outermost layers of the skin and hair. An example of a fungal infection is Tinea versicolor: Tinea versicolor is a fungus infection that commonly affects the skin of young people, especially the chest, back, and upper arms and legs.

Mycosis fungoides	Mycosis fungoides, is the most common form of cutaneous T-cell lymphoma. It generally affects the skin, but may progress internally over time. Mycosis fungoides was first described in 1806 by French dermatologist Jean-Louis-Marc Alibert.
Breastfeeding	Suckling and nursing are synonyms. For other uses, see Nursing (disambiguation) and Suckling (disambiguation) breastfeeding is the feeding of an infant or young child with breast milk directly from human breasts (i.e., via lactation) rather than from a baby bottle or other container. Babies have a sucking reflex that enables them to suck and swallow milk.
Genitourinary system	In anatomy, the Genitourinary system or urogenital system is the organ system of the reproductive organs and the urinary system. These are grouped together because of their proximity to each other, their common embryological origin and the use of common pathways, like the male urethra. Also, because of their proximity, the systems are sometimes imaged together.
Kidney	The kidneys are paired organs, which have the production of urine as their primary function. kidneys are seen in many types of animals, including vertebrates and some invertebrates. They are an essential part of the urinary system, but have several secondary functions concerned with homeostatic functions.
Wound healing	Wound healing, or wound repair, is an intricate process in which the skin (or some other organ) repairs itself after injury. In normal skin, the epidermis (outermost layer) and dermis (inner or deeper layer) exists in a steady-state equilibrium, forming a protective barrier against the external environment. Once the protective barrier is broken, the normal (physiologic) process of wound healing is immediately set in motion.
Nosocomial	Nosocomial infections are infections which are a result of treatment in a hospital or a healthcare service unit, but not secondary to the patient`s original condition. Infections are considered nosocomial if they first appear 48 hours or more after hospital admission or within 30 days after discharge. nosocomial comes from the Greek word nosokomeion meaning hospital (nosos = disease, komeo = to take care of).

Chapter 3. PART III: Chapter 5 - Chapter 6

Circulatory system	The circulatory system is an organ system that passes nutrients (such as amino acids and electrolytes), gases, hormones, blood cells, etc. to and from cells in the body to help fight diseases and help stabilize body temperature and pH to maintain homeostasis. This system may be seen strictly as a blood distribution network, but some consider the circulatory system as composed of the cardiovascular system, which distributes blood, and the lymphatic system, which distributes lymph.
Body fluid	Body fluid or bodily fluids are liquids that are inside the bodies of living organisms. They include fluids that are excreted or secreted from the body as well as body water that normally is not. · Amniotic fluid surrounding a fetus · Cerebrospinal fluid · Cowper's fluid or pre-ejaculatory fluid · Chyme · Blood · Blood plasma · Serum · Extracellular fluid · Aqueous humour · Lymph · Female ejaculate · Interstitial fluid · Pleural fluid · Pus

· Urine

· Vomit

Body secretions include:

· Cerumen also known as earwax

· Gastric juice

· Breast milk

· Mucus (including nasal drainage and phlegm)

· Saliva

· Sebum (skin oil)

· Semen

· Sweat

· Tears

· Vaginal secretion

Bodily fluids are regarded with varying levels of disgust among world cultures, including the Abrahamic faiths (Christianity, Islam, Judaism) and Hinduism. In Hinduism substances that have left the body are considered unclean, although there are some alleged consumption of some ancient sects of the urine of people.

Routes	Routes is a commune in the Seine-Maritime department in the Haute-Normandie region in northern France.
Vertigo	Vertigo) is a type of dizziness, where there is a feeling of motion when one is stationary. The symptoms are due to a dysfunction of the vestibular system in the inner ear. It is often associated with nausea and vomiting as well as difficulties standing or walking.

Hypotension	In physiology and medicine, hypotension is abnormally low blood pressure. This is best understood as a physiologic state, rather than a disease. It is often associated with shock, though not necessarily indicative of it.
Orthostatic hypotension	Orthostatic hypotension (also known as postural hypotension orthostasis, and, colloquially, as head rush or a dizzy spell and to some people `the elevator effect`) is a form of hypotension in which a person`s blood pressure suddenly falls when the person stands up. The decrease is typically greater than 20/10 mm Hg, and may be most pronounced after resting. The incidence increases with age.
Prostate	The prostate is a compound tubuloalveolar exocrine gland of the male reproductive system in most mammals. Females do not have prostate glands. A gland in females with similar characteristics to the prostate, previously called paraurethral or Skene`s glands, connected to the distal third of the urethra in the prevaginal space has been considered by a few researchers as a `prostate-like` gland.
Prostheses	In medicine, a prosthesis is an artificial extension that replaces a missing body part. It is part of the field of biomechatronics, the science of using mechanical devices with human muscle, skeleton, and nervous systems to assist or enhance motor control lost by trauma, disease, or defect. prostheses are typically used to replace parts lost by injury or missing from birth (congenital) or to supplement defective body parts.
Walker	A walker is a tool for disabled or elderly people who need additional support to maintain balance or stability while walking. The British English common equivalent term for a walker is Zimmer frame - from Zimmer Holdings, a major manufacturer of such devices and joint replacement parts. A type of walker was patented on 10 May 1988 by Andrejs Muiza who immigrated to the United States (Nashville, TN) from Latvia following World War II. The basic design consists of a frame that is about waist high, approximately twelve inches deep and slightly wider than the user.
Epiglottitis	Epiglottitis is inflammation of the epiglottis - the flap that sits at the base of the tongue, which keeps food from going into the trachea (windpipe). Due to its place in the airway, swelling of this structure can interfere with breathing and constitutes a medical emergency. The infection can cause the epiglottis to either obstruct or completely close off the windpipe.

Chickenpox	Chickenpox or chicken pox is a highly contagious illness caused by primary infection with varicella zoster virus (VZV). It usually starts with vesicular skin rash mainly on the body and head rather than at the periphery and become itchy raw pockmarks which mostly heal without scarring. Chicken pox is spread easily through coughs or sneezes of ill individuals, or through direct contact with secretions from the rash.
Violence	Violence is the expression of physical or verbal force against self or other, compelling action against one`s will on pain of being hurt. Worldwide, violence is used as a tool of manipulation and also is an area of concern for law and culture which take attempts to suppress and stop it. The word violence covers a broad spectrum.
Bronchopneumonia	Bronchopneumonia or bronchial pneumonia (also known as lobular pneumonia) is a type of pneumonia characterized by multiple foci of isolated, acute consolidation, affecting one or more pulmonary lobes. It is one of two types of bacterial pneumonia as classified by gross anatomic distribution of consolidation (solidification), the other being lobar pneumonia. Bronchopneumonia is less likely than lobar pneumonia to be associated with Streptococcus.
Tracheostomy	Tracheotomy and Tracheostomy are surgical procedures on the neck to open a direct airway through an incision in the trachea (the windpipe). They are performed by paramedics, veterinarians, emergency physicians and surgeons. Both surgical and percutaneous techniques are now widely used.
Lithotomy position	The lithotomy position is a medical term referring to a common position for surgical procedures and medical examinations involving the pelvis and lower abdomen, as well as a common position for childbirth in Western nations. The lithotomy position involves the positioning of an individual's feet above or at the same level as the hips (often in stirrups), with the perineum positioned at the edge of an examination table. References to the position have been found in some of the oldest known medical documents including versions of the Hippocratic oath ; the position is named after the ancient surgical procedure for removing kidney stones, gall stones and bladder stones via the perineum. The position is perhaps most recognizable as the 'often used' position for childbirth: the patient is laid on the back with knees bent, positioned above the hips, and spread apart through the use of stirrups

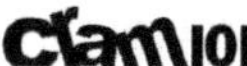

Supine position	The Supine position is a position of the body: lying down with the face up, as opposed to the prone position, which is face down, sometimes with the hands behind the head or neck. When used in surgical procedures, it allows access to the peritoneal, thoracic and pericardial regions; as well as the head, neck and extremities. Using terms defined in the anatomical position, the dorsal side is down, and the ventral side is up.
Trendelenburg position	In the Trendelenburg position the body is laid flat on the back (supine position) with the feet higher than the head, in contrast to the reverse Trendelenburg position, where the body is tilted in the opposite direction. This is a standard position used in abdominal and gynecological surgery. It allows better access to the pelvic organs as gravity pulls the intestines away from the pelvis.
Sildenafil	Sildenafil citrate, sold as Viagra, Revatio and under various other trade names, is a drug used to treat erectile dysfunction and pulmonary arterial hypertension (PAH). It was developed and is being marketed by the pharmaceutical company Pfizer. It acts by inhibiting cGMP specific phosphodiesterase type 5, an enzyme that regulates blood flow in the penis.
Frequency	Frequency is the number of occurrences of a repeating event per unit time. It is also referred to as temporal frequency. The period is the duration of one cycle in a repeating event, so the period is the reciprocal of the frequency.
Hyperactivity	Hyperactivity can be described as a physical state in which a person is abnormally and easily excitable or exuberant. Strong emotional reactions, impulsive behavior, and sometimes a short span of attention are also typical for a hyperactive person. Some individuals may show these characteristics naturally, as personality differs from person to person.
REM sleep	Rapid Eye Movement (REM) sleep is a normal stage of sleep characterized by the rapid movement of the eyes. REM sleep is classified into two categories: tonic and phasic. It was identified and defined by Kleitman and Aserinsky in the early 1950s.
Sleep deprivation	Sleep deprivation is the condition of not having enough sleep; it can be either chronic or acute. A chronic sleep-restricted state can cause fatigue, daytime sleepiness, clumsiness and weight loss or weight gain. It adversely affects the brain and cognitive function.
Sedative	A sedative is a substance that induces sedation by reducing irritability or excitement.

	At higher doses it may result in slurred speech, staggering gait, poor judgment, and slow, uncertain reflexes. Doses of sedatives such as benzodiazepines when used as a hypnotic to induce sleep tend to be higher than those used to relieve anxiety whereas only low doses are needed to provide calming sedative effects.
Sedentary lifestyle	Sedentary lifestyle is a medical term used to denote a type of lifestyle with a no or irregular physical activity. It is commonly found in both the developed and developing world and characterized by sitting, reading, watching television and computer use for much of the day with little or no vigorous physical exercise. It is known to contribute to obesity and cardiovascular disease.
Liver	The liver is a vital organ present in vertebrates and some other animals. It has a wide range of functions, including detoxification, protein synthesis, and production of biochemicals necessary for digestion. The liver is necessary for survival; there is currently no way to compensate for the absence of liver function.
Health education	Health education is the profession of educating people about health. Areas within this profession encompass environmental health, physical health, social health, emotional health, intellectual health, and spiritual health. It can be defined as the principle by which individuals and groups of people learn to behave in a manner conducive to the promotion, maintenance, or restoration of health.
Self-efficacy	Self-efficacy has been described as the belief that one is capable of performing in a certain manner to attain certain goals. It is a belief that one has the capabilities to execute the courses of actions required to manage prospective situations. It has been described in other ways as the concept has evolved in the literature and in society: as the sense of belief that one\`s actions have an effect on the environment ; as a person\`s judgment of his or her capabilities based on mastery criteria; a sense of a person\`s competence within a specific framework, focusing on the person\`s assessment of their abilities to perform specific tasks in relation to goals and standards rather than in comparison with others\` capabilities.
Range of motion	Range of motion or , is the distance (linear or angular) that a movable object may normally travel while properly attached to another object. It is also called range of travel, particularly when talking about mechanical devices and in mechanical engineering fields. For example, a volume knob (a rotary fader) may have a 300° range of travel from the \`off\` or muted (fully attenuated) position at lower left, going clockwise to its maximum-loudness position at lower right.

Chapter 3. PART III: Chapter 5 - Chapter 6

Gait	Gait is the pattern of movement of the limbs of terrestrial animals, including humans, during locomotion. Most animals use a variety of gaits, selecting gait based on speed, terrain, the need to maneuver, and energetic efficiency. Different animal species may use different gaits due to differences in anatomy that prevent use of certain gaits, or simply due to evolved innate preferences as a result of habitat differences.
Informed consent	Informed consent is a legal condition whereby a person can be said to have given consent based upon a clear appreciation and understanding of the facts, implications and future consequences of an action. In order to give Informed consent, the individual concerned must have adequate reasoning faculties and be in possession of all relevant facts at the time consent is given. Impairments to reasoning and judgement which would make it impossible for someone to give Informed consent include such factors as severe mental retardation, severe mental illness, intoxication, severe sleep deprivation, Alzheimer`s disease, or being in a coma.
Carbohydrate	A carbohydrate is an organic compound with general formula $C_m(H_2O)_n$, that is, consisting only of carbon, hydrogen and oxygen, the last two in the 2:1 atom ratio. carbohydrates can be viewed as hydrates of carbon, hence their name. The term is most commonly used in biochemistry, where it is essentially a synonym of saccharide, a large family of natural carbohydrates that fill numerous roles in living things, such as the storage and transport of energy (e.g., starch, glycogen), structural components (e.g., cellulose in plants and chitin in arthropods), and as components of coenzymes (e.g., ATP, FAD, and NAD) and the backbone of genetic molecules (e.g., RNA and DNA).
Protein	Proteins (also known as polypeptides) are organic compounds made of amino acids arranged in a linear chain and folded into a globular form. The amino acids in a polymer are joined together by the peptide bonds between the carboxyl and amino groups of adjacent amino acid residues. The sequence of amino acids in a protein is defined by the sequence of a gene, which is encoded in the genetic code.
Lactose	Lactose is a sugar that is found most notably in milk. lactose makes up around 2-8% of milk (by weight), although the amount varies among species and individuals. It is extracted from sweet or sour whey.

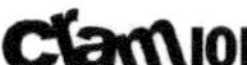

Lactose intolerance	Lactose intolerance is the inability to metabolize lactose, because of a lack of the required enzyme lactase in the digestive system. It is estimated that 75% of adults worldwide show some decrease in lactase activity during adulthood. The frequency of decreased lactase activity ranges from as little as 5% in northern Europe, up to 71% for Sicily, to more than 90% in some African and Asian countries. There are three major types of lactose intolerance: · Primary lactose intolerance.
Anorexia	Anorexia is the decreased sensation of appetite. While the term in non-scientific publications is often used interchangeably with Anorexia nervosa, many possible causes exist for a decreased appetite, some of which may be harmless, while others indicate a serious clinical condition, or pose a significant risk.
Taste	Taste (or, more formally, gustation) is a form of direct chemoreception and is one of the traditional five senses. It refers to the ability to detect the flavor of substances such as food, certain minerals, and poisons. In humans and many other vertebrate animals the sense of taste partners with the less direct sense of smell, in the brain`s perception of flavor.
Sense	Senses are the physiological methods of perception. The Senses and their operation, classification, and theory are overlapping topics studied by a variety of fields, most notably neuroscience, cognitive psychology (or cognitive science), and philosophy of perception. The nervous system has a specific sensory system, or organ, dedicated to each Sense.
Occupational therapy	Occupational therapy, often abbreviated as , uses meaningful and purposeful occupations to promote health. These can be work related activities to leisure activities. Occupational therapists work with individuals, families, groups and communities to facilitate health and well-being through engagement or re-engagement in occupation.
Oral stage	The Oral stage in psychoanalysis is the term used by Sigmund Freud to describe his theory of child development during the first 21 months of life, in which an infant`s pleasure centers are in the mouth. This is the first of Freud`s psychosexual stages. In Freud`s theory, this is the infant`s first relationship with its mother; it is a nutritive one.

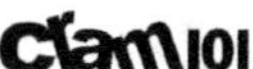

Cranial nerves	Cranial nerves are nerves that emerge directly from the brain stem, in contrast to spinal nerves which emerge from segments of the spinal cord. Human Cranial nerves are evolutionarily homologous to those found in many other vertebrates. Cranial nerves XI and XII evolved in the common ancestor to amniotes (non-amphibian tetrapods) thus totaling twelve pairs.
Apraxia	Apraxia is a neurological disorder characterized by loss of the ability to execute or carry out learned purposeful movements, despite having the desire and the physical ability to perform the movements. It is a disorder of motor planning which may be acquired or developmental, but may not be caused by incoordination, sensory loss, or failure to comprehend simple commands . Apraxia should not be confused with aphasia, an inability to produce and/or comprehend language, abulia, the lack of desire to carry out an action, or allochiria, in which patients perceive stimuli to one side of the body as occurring on the other.
Enteral	Enteral is a term used to describe the intestines or other portions of the digestive tract. This is contrasted with parEnteral, or non-digestive, system methods of introducing drugs or substances into the body, via, for example, injection. It includes oral, rectal, and sublingual administration as a route of administration for drugs.
Delusion	A delusion is a fixed belief that is either false, fanciful, or derived from deception. In psychiatry, it is defined to be a belief that is pathological (the result of an illness or illness process) and is held despite evidence to the contrary. As a pathology, it is distinct from a belief based on false or incomplete information, dogma, stupidity, apperception, illusion, or other effects of perception.
Joint replacement	Joint replacement surgery is a procedure of orthopedic surgery, in which the arthritic or dysfunctional joint surface is replaced with an orthopaedic prosthesis. Join replacement is considered as a treatment when severe joint pain or dysfunction is not alleviated by less-invasive therapies.
Rape	Rape, also referred to as sexual assault, is an assault by a person involving sexual intercourse with or without sexual penetration of another person without that person`s consent.

The rate of reporting, prosecution and convictions f varies considerably in different jurisdictions. The U.S. Bureau of Justice Statistics (1999) estimated that 91% of U.S. rape victims are female and 9% are male, with 99% of the offenders being male.

Crisis intervention

Crisis intervention can be defined as emergency psychological care aimed to assist individuals in returning to normal levels of functioning and to prevent or alleviate potential negative psychological trauma . Crisis can be defined as one's perception or experiencing of an event or situation as an intolerable difficulty that exceeds the person's current resources and coping mechanisms. The priority of Crisis intervention/counseling is to increase stabilization.

Symptom

A symptom is a departure from normal function or feeling which is noticed by a patient, indicating the presence of disease or abnormality. A symptom is subjective, observed by the patient, and not measured.
symptoms may be chronic, relapsing or remitting.

Rape trauma syndrome

Rape Trauma Syndrome is a form of psychological trauma and post traumatic stress disorder experienced by a rape victim, consisting of disruptions to normal physical, emotional, cognitive, behavioral, and interpersonal characteristics. The theory was first described by psychiatrist Ann Wolbert Burgess and sociologist Lynda Lytle Holmstrom in 1974.

Rape trauma syndrome describes a cluster of psychological and physical signs, symptoms and reactions common to most rape victims, during, immediately following, and for months or years after a rape.

Psychosis

Psychosis literally means abnormal condition of the mind, and is a generic psychiatric term for a mental state often described as involving a `loss of contact with reality`. People suffering from psychosis are said to be psychotic.

People experiencing psychosis may report hallucinations or delusional beliefs, and may exhibit personality changes and thought disorder.

Headache

In medicine a headache or cephalalgia is a symptom of a number of different conditions of the head. headache is caused by a disturbance of the pain-sensitive structures in the head. The brain in itself is not sensitive to pain, because it lacks nociceptors.

Somatic	The term somatic refers to cells of the body, rather than gametes . In humans, somatic cells contain two copies of each chromosome (diploid), whereas gametes only contain one copy of each chromosome (haploid). Although all somatic cells of an individual are genetically identical in principle, they evolve a variety of tissue-specific characteristics during the process of differentiation, through epigenetic and regulatory alterations.
Locus of control	Locus of control is a term in psychology that refers to a person`s belief about what causes the good or bad results in his life, either in general or in a specific area such as health or academics. Understanding of the concept was developed by Julian B. Rotter in 1954, and has since become an important aspect of personality studies. Locus of control refers to the extent to which individuals believe that they can control events that affect them.
Colostomy	A Colostomy is a surgical procedure that involves connecting a part of the colon onto the anterior abdominal wall, leaving the patient with an opening on the abdomen called a stoma. In a Colostomy, the stoma is formed from the end of the large intestine, which is drawn out through the incision and sutured to the skin. After a Colostomy, feces leave the patient's body through the abdomen.
Epidermis	The epidermis is the outer layer of the skin, composed of terminally differentiated stratified squamous epithelium, acting as the body`s major barrier against an inhospitable environment. It is the thinnest on the eyelids at .05 mm (0.0020 in) and the thickest on the palms and soles at 1.5 mm (0.059 in). It is ectodermal in origin.
Collagen	Collagen is the main protein of connective tissue in animals and the most abundant protein in mammals, making up about 25% to 35% of the whole-body protein content. It is naturally found exclusively in metazoa, including sponges. In muscle tissue it serves as a major component of endomysium.
Pallor	Pallor is a reduced amount of oxyhemoglobin in skin or mucous membrane, a pale color which can be caused by illness, emotional shock or stress, avoiding excessive exposure to sunlight, anemia or genetics. It is more evident on the face and palms. It can develop suddenly or gradually, depending on the cause.

Contact lenses

A contact lens (also known simply as a contact) is a corrective, cosmetic, or therapeutic lens usually placed on the cornea of the eye. Leonardo da Vinci is credited with describing and sketching the first ideas f in 1508, but it was more than 300 years later before Contact lenses were actually fabricated and worn on the eye. Modern soft Contact lenses were invented by the Czech chemist Otto Wichterle and his assistant Drahoslav Lím, who also invented the first gel used for their production.

Nitrogen balance

Nitrogen balance is the measure of nitrogen output subtracted from nitrogen input.

Blood urea nitrogen can be used in estimating Nitrogen balance, as can the urea concentration in urine.

A positive value is often found during periods of growth, tissue repair or pregnancy.

Oral hygiene

Oral hygiene is the practice of keeping the mouth and teeth clean to prevent dental problems and bad breath. class="rellink boilerplate seealso">.

Mucositis

Mucositis is the painful inflammation and ulceration of the mucous membranes lining the digestive tract, usually as an adverse effect of chemotherapy and radiotherapy treatment for cancer. Mucositis can occur anywhere along the gastrointestinal (GI) tract, but oral Mucositis refers to the particular inflammation and ulceration that occurs in the mouth. Oral Mucositis is a common and often debilitating complication of cancer treatment.

Stomatitis

Stomatitis is an inflammation of the mucous lining of any of the structures in the mouth, which may involve the cheeks, gums, tongue, lips, throat, and roof or floor of the mouth. The inflammation can be caused by conditions in the mouth itself, such as poor oral hygiene, poorly fitted dentures, or from mouth burns from hot food or drinks, toxic plants,or by conditions that affect the entire body, such as medications, allergic reactions, radiation therapy, or infections.

Teeth

Teeth are small, calcified, whitish structures found in the jaws (or mouths) of many vertebrates that are used to tear, scrape, and chew food. Some animals, particularly carnivores, also use teeth for hunting or defense. The roots of teeth are covered by gums.

Consciousness

Consciousness is variously defined as subjective experience, or awareness, or wakefulness, or the executive control system of the mind. It is an umbrella term that may refer to a variety of mental phenomena. Although humans realize what everyday experiences are, Consciousness refuses to be defined, philosophers note :

	Consciousness in medicine (e.g., anesthesiology) is assessed by observing a patient's alertness and responsiveness, and can be seen as a continuum of states ranging from alert, oriented to time and place, and communicative, through disorientation, then delirium, then loss of any meaningful communication, and ending with loss of movement in response to painful stimulation.
Long-term care	Long-term care (LTC) is a variety of services which help meet both the medical and non-medical need of people with a chronic illness or disability who cannot care for themselves for long periods of time. It is common f to provide custodial and non-skilled care, such as assisting with normal daily tasks like dressing, bathing, and using the bathroom. Increasingly, long term care involves providing a level of medical care that requires the expertise of skilled practitioners to address the often multiple chronic conditions associated with older populations.
Myocardial infarction	Myocardial infarction or acute myocardial infarction (AMI), commonly known as a heart attack, is the interruption of blood supply to part of the heart, causing some heart cells to die. This is most commonly due to occlusion (blockage) of a coronary artery following the rupture of a vulnerable atherosclerotic plaque, which is an unstable collection of lipids (fatty acids) and white blood cells (especially macrophages) in the wall of an artery. The resulting ischemia (restriction in blood supply) and oxygen shortage, if left untreated for a sufficient period of time, can cause damage or death (infarction) of heart muscle tissue (myocardium).
Infarction	In medicine, an Infarction is the formation of an infarct, that is, an area of tissue death (necrosis) due to a local lack of oxygen caused by obstruction of the tissue`s blood supply.. The supplying artery may be blocked by an obstruction , may be mechanically compressed (e.g. tumor, volvulus, or hernia), ruptured by trauma (e.g. atherosclerosis or vasculitides), or vasoconstricted (e.g. cocaine vasoconstriction leading to myocardial Infarction). Hypertension and atherosclerosis are risk factors for both atherosclerotic plaques and thromboembolism.
Premature infant	In humans, preterm birth refers to the birth of a baby of less than 37 weeks gestational age. Premature birth, commonly used as a synonym for preterm birth, refers to the birth of a Premature infant. The child may commonly be referred to throughout their life as being born a `preemie` or `preemie baby`.

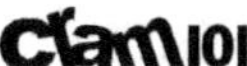

Hypoventilation	In medicine, Hypoventilation occurs when ventilation is inadequate (hypo means `below`) to perform needed gas exchange. By definition it causes an increased concentration of carbon dioxide (hypercapnia) and respiratory acidosis. It can be caused by medical conditions, such as stroke affecting the brainstem, by holding one`s breath, or by drugs, typically when taken in overdose.
Vital signs	Vital signs are measures of various physiological statistics, often taken by health professionals, in order to assess the most basic body functions. vital signs are an essential part of a case presentation. The act of taking vital signs normally entails recording Body temperature, Pulse rate (or heart rate), Blood pressure, and Respiratory rate, but may also include other measurements.
Airway resistance	Airway resistance is a concept used in respiratory physiology to describe mechanical factors which limit the access of inspired air to the pulmonary alveoli, and thus determine airflow. Resistance is greatest at the bronchi of intermediate size, in between the fourth and eighth bifurcation. Because Airway resistance is dictated by the diameter of the airways and by the density of the inspired gas, the low density of heliox reduces Airway resistance, and makes it easier to ventilate the lungs.
Hypoxemia	Hypoxemia is generally defined as decreased partial pressure of oxygen in blood, sometimes specifically as less than 60 mmHg (8.0 kPa) or causing hemoglobin oxygen saturation of less than 90%. The hypoxemia definition as decreased partial pressure of oxygen excludes decreased oxygen content caused by anemia (decreased content of oxygen binding protein hemoglobin) or other primary hemoglobin deficiency, because they don`t decrease the partial pressure of oxygen in blood. Still, some simply define it as insufficient oxygenation or total oxygen content of (arterial) blood, which, without further specification, would include both concentration of dissolved oxygen and oxygen bound to hemoglobin.

Intracranial pressure	Intracranial pressure is the pressure in the cranium and thus in the brain tissue and cerebrospinal fluid (CSF); this pressure is exerted on the brain`s intracranial blood circulation vessels. ICP is maintained in a tight normal range dynamically, through the production and absorption of CSF and pulsates approximately 1mm Hg in a normal healthy adult. CSF pressure has been shown to be influenced by abrupt changes in intrathoracic pressure during coughing (intraabdominal pressure), valsalva (Queckenstedt`s maneuver), and communication with the vasculature (venous and arterial systems).
Weakness	Weakness is a symptom used to describe a number of different conditions, including: lack of muscle strength, malaise, dizziness or fatigue. The causes are many and can be divided into conditions that have true or perceived muscle weakness. True muscle weakness is a primary symptom of a variety of skeletal muscle diseases, including muscular dystrophy and inflammatory myopathy.
Dressing	A dressing is an adjunct used by a person for application to a wound to promote healing and/or prevent further harm. A dressing is designed to be in direct contact with the wound, which makes it different from a bandage, which is primarily used to hold a dressing in place. Some organisations classify them as the same thing (for example, the British Pharmacopoeia) and the terms are used interchangeably by some people.
Hysterectomy	A hysterectomy is the surgical removal of the uterus, usually performed by a gynecologist. hysterectomy may be total or partial (removal of the uterine body but leaving the cervical stump, also called `supracervical`). It is the most commonly performed gynecological surgical procedure.
Bulimia	Bulimia nervosa is an eating disorder characterized by recurrent binge eating, followed by compensatory behaviors. The most common form is defensive vomiting, sometimes called purging; fasting, the use of laxatives, enemas, diuretics, and over exercising are also common. The word Bulimia derives from the Latin , which originally comes from the Greek βουλιμΐ¯α (boulÄ«mia; ravenous hunger), a compound of βους (bous), ox + λιμΪŒς (lÄ«mos), hunger.
Bulimia nervosa	Bulimia nervosa is an eating disorder characterized by recurrent binge eating, followed by compensatory behaviors. The most common form is defensive vomiting, sometimes called purging; fasting, the use of laxatives, enemas, diuretics, and over exercising are also common. The word bulimia derives from the Latin , which originally comes from the Greek βουλιμΐ¯α (boulÄ«mia; ravenous hunger), a compound of βους (bous), ox + λιμΪŒς (lÄ«mos), hunger.

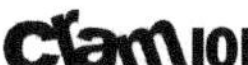

Haemophilus influenzae	Haemophilus influenzae, formerly called Pfeiffer`s bacillus or Bacillus influenzae, is a non-motile Gram-negative rod-shaped bacterium first described in 1892 by Richard Pfeiffer during an influenza pandemic. A member of the Pasteurellaceae family, it is generally aerobic, but can grow as a facultative anaerobe. H. influenzae was mistakenly considered to be the cause of influenza until 1933, when the viral etiology of the flu became apparent.
Chemotherapy	Chemotherapy, in its most general sense, is the treatment of disease by chemicals especially by killing micro-organisms or cancerous cells. In popular usage, it refers to antineoplastic drugs used to treat cancer or the combination of these drugs into a cytotoxic standardized treatment regimen. In its non-oncological use, the term may also refer to antibiotics (antibacterial chemotherapy).
Hormone	A hormone is a chemical released by one or more cells that affects cells in other parts of the organism. Only a small amount of hormone is required to alter cell metabolism. It is essentially a chemical messenger that transports a signal from one cell to another.
Vitamin	A Vitamin is an organic compound required as a nutrient in tiny amounts by an organism. The term Vitamin was derived from `Vitamine,` a combination word from vita and amine, meaning amine of life, because it was suggested that the organic micronutrient food factors which prevented beriberi and perhaps other similar dietary-deficiency diseases, might be chemical amines. This proved incorrect for the micronutrient class, and the word was shortened.
Hallucination	A Hallucination, in the broadest sense, is a perception in the absence of a stimulus. In a stricter sense, Hallucinations are defined as perceptions in a conscious and awake state in the absence of external stimuli which have qualities of real perception, in that they are vivid, substantial, and located in external objective space. The latter definition distinguishes Hallucinations from the related phenomena of dreaming, which does not involve wakefulness; illusion, which involves distorted or misinterpreted real perception; imagery, which does not mimic real perception and is under voluntary control; and pseudoHallucination, which does not mimic real perception, but is not under voluntary control.
Schizophrenia	Schizophrenia is a mental disorder characterized by a disintegration of thought processes and of emotional responsiveness. It most commonly manifests as auditory hallucinations, paranoid or bizarre delusions, or disorganized speech and thinking, and it is accompanied by significant social or occupational dysfunction. The onset of symptoms typically occurs in young adulthood, with a global lifetime prevalence of about 0.3-0.7%.

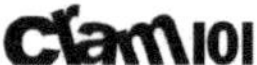

Reframing	The term Reframing designates a communication technique which has origins in family systems therapy and the work of Virginia Satir. Milton H. Erickson has been associated with Reframing and it also forms an important part of Neuro-linguistic programming. In addition, provocative therapy uses Reframing with an emphasis on humor.
Risk assessment	Risk assessment is a step in a risk management process. risk assessment is the determination of quantitative or qualitative value of risk related to a concrete situation and a recognized threat (also called hazard). Quantitative risk assessment requires calculations of two components of risk: R, the magnitude of the potential loss L, and the probability p, that the loss will occur.
Suicide prevention	Suicide prevention is an umbrella term for the collective efforts of local citizen organizations, mental health practitioners and related professionals to reduce the incidence of suicide through pre-vention and proactive measures. One of the first exclusively professional research centers was established 1958 in Los Angeles. The first crisis hotline service in the U.S. run by selected, trained citizen volunteers was established 1961 in San Francisco. Various suicide prevention strategies have been used: · Selection and training of volunteer citizen groups offering confidential referral services. · Promoting mental resilience through optimism and connectedness. · Education about suicide, including risk factors, warning signs and the availability of help. · Increasing the proficiency of health and welfare services at responding to people in need.
Sexual dysfunction	Sexual dysfunction or sexual malfunction refers to a difficulty experienced by an individual or a couple during any stage of a normal sexual activity, including desire, arousal or orgasm. sexual dysfunction disorders may be classified into four categories: sexual desire disorders, arousal disorders, orgasm disorders and pain disorders. Sexual desire disorders or decreased libido are characterised by a lack or absence for some period of time of sexual desire or libido for sexual activity or of sexual fantasies.

Sexual assault	Sexual assault is an assault of a sexual nature on another person. Although sexual assaults most frequently are by a man on a woman, it may be by a man on a man, woman on a man or woman on a woman, and man or woman on a child. Approximately one in six American women will be a victim of a sexual assault in her lifetime.
Group psychotherapy	Group psychotherapy is a form of psychotherapy in which one or more therapists treat a small group of clients together as a group. The term can legitimately refer to any form of psychotherapy when delivered in a group format, including Cognitive behavioural therapy or Interpersonal therapy, but it is usually applied to psychodynamic group therapy where the group context and group process is explicitly utilised as a mechanism of change by developing, exploring and examining interpersonal relationships within the group. The broader concept of group therapy can be taken to include any helping process that takes place in a group, including support groups, skills training groups (such as anger management, mindfulness, relaxation training or social skills training), and psycho-education groups.
Pelvic	In human anatomy, the pelvis is the part of the trunk inferioposterior to the abdomen in the transition area between the trunk and the lower limbs. The term is used to denote several structures: · the Pelvic girdle or bony pelvis, the irregular ring-shaped bony structure connecting the spine to the femurs, · the Pelvic cavity, the space enclosed by the Pelvic girdle, subdivided into · the greater or false pelvis (inferior part of the abdominal cavity) and · the lesser or true pelvis which provides the skeletal framework for the perineum and the Pelvic cavity (which are separated by the Pelvic diaphragm), · the Pelvic region. \`Pelvis\` is the Latin word for a \`basin\` and the pelvis thus got its name from its shape. It is also known as hip girdle or coxa girdle.

Pelvic floor	The pelvic floor or pelvic diaphragm is composed of muscle fibers of the levator ani, the coccygeus, and associated connective tissue which span the area underneath the pelvis. The pelvic diaphragm is a muscular partition formed by the levatores ani and coccygei, with which may be included the parietal pelvic fascia on their upper and lower aspects. The pelvic floor separates the pelvic cavity above from the perineal region (including perineum) below.
Prayer	Prayer is a form of religious practice that seeks to activate a volitional connection to some greater power in the universe through deliberate intentional practice. prayer may be either individual or communal and take place in public or in private. It may involve the use of words, song, or complete silence.
Faith	Faith is the confident belief or trust in the truth or trustworthiness of a person, concept or thing. The English word is thought to date from 1200-50, from the Latin fidem or fidÄ"s, meaning trust, derived from the verb fÄ«dere, to trust. The term is employed in a religious or theological context to refer to a confident belief in a transcendent reality, a religious teacher, a set of scriptures, teachings or a Supreme Being.
Respiratory therapy	Respiratory therapy is an allied health field involved in the assessment and treatment of breathing disorders including chronic lung problems (i.e., asthma , bronchitis , emphysema , COPD) ,and more acute multi systemic problems stemming from other pathological conditions such as heart attacks, strokes, shock, asphyxiation, drowning shock or trauma. Respiratory Therapists are specialists in airway management, mechanical ventilation, acid/base balance and critical care medicine. A thorough education in anatomy, physiology, pathophysiology, pharmaceutical agents, chemistry, physics, hemodynamics, and mechanical ventilation enables the Respiratory therapy to function as an indispensable member of the health care team.
Palliative care	Palliative care is any form of medical care or treatment that concentrates on reducing the severity of disease symptoms, rather than striving to halt, delay, or reverse progression of the disease itself or provide a cure. The goal is to prevent and relieve suffering and to improve quality of life for people facing serious, complex illness. Non-hospice palliative care is not dependent on prognosis and is offered in conjunction with curative and all other appropriate forms of medical treatment.

Religiosity	Religiosity, in its broadest sense, is a comprehensive sociological term used to refer to the numerous aspects of religious activity, dedication, and belief (religious doctrine). Another term that would work equally well, though is less often used, is religiousness. In its narrowest sense, Religiosity deals more with how religious a person is, and less with how a person is religious (in practicing certain rituals, retelling certain myths, revering certain symbols, or accepting certain doctrines about deities and afterlife).
Sudden infant death syndrome	Sudden infant death syndrome or crib death is a syndrome marked by the sudden death of an infant that is unexpected by history and remains unexplained after a thorough forensic autopsy and a detailed death scene investigation. The term cot death is often used in the United Kingdom, Ireland, Australia, India, South Africa and New Zealand. Typically the infant is found dead after having been put to bed, and exhibits no signs of having suffered.
Cardiovascular system	The circulatory system is an organ system that passes nutrients (such as amino acids and electrolytes), gases, hormones, blood cells etc. to and from cells in the body to help fight diseases and help stabilize body temperature and pH to maintain homeostasis. This system may be seen strictly as a blood distribution network, but some consider the circulatory system as composed of the cardiovascular system, which distributes blood, and the lymphatic system, which distributes lymph.
Esophageal varices	In medicine (gastroenterology), esophageal varices are extremely dilated sub-mucosal veins in the lower esophagus. They are most often a consequence of portal hypertension, commonly due to cirrhosis; patients with esophageal varices have a strong tendency to develop bleeding. esophageal varices are diagnosed with endoscopy.
Varicella	Chickenpox or chicken pox is a highly contagious illness caused by primary infection with varicella zoster virus (VZV). It usually starts with vesicular skin rash mainly on the body and head rather than at the periphery and become itchy raw pockmarks which mostly heal without scarring. Chicken pox is spread easily through coughs or sneezes of ill individuals, or through direct contact with secretions from the rash.

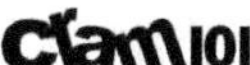

Thrombosis	Thrombosis is the formation of a blood clot (thrombus) inside a blood vessel, obstructing the flow of blood through the circulatory system. When a blood vessel is injured, the body uses platelets and fibrin to form a blood clot, because the first step in repairing it (hemostasis) is to prevent loss of blood. If that mechanism causes too much clotting, and the clot breaks free, an embolus is formed.
Atherosclerosis	Atherosclerosis is the condition in which an artery wall thickens as the result of a build-up of fatty materials such as cholesterol. It is a syndrome affecting arterial blood vessels, a chronic inflammatory response in the walls of arteries, in large part due to the accumulation of macrophage white blood cells and promoted by Low-density lipoproteins (plasma proteins that carry cholesterol and triglycerides) without adequate removal of fats and cholesterol from the macrophages by functional high density lipoproteins (HDL), . It is commonly referred to as a hardening or furring of the arteries.
Enuresis	Enuresis refers to an inability to control urination. Use of the term is usually limited to describing individuals old enough to be expected to exercise such control. Types include: · Nocturnal Enuresis · Diurnal Enuresis .
Urinary retention	Urinary retention also known as ischuria is a lack of ability to urinate. It is a common complication of benign prostatic hypertrophy (also known as benign prostatic hyperplasia or BPH), although anticholinergics may also play a role, and requires a catheter or prostatic stent. Various pharmaceuticals can cause Urinary retention, including some antidepressants, COX-2 inhibitors, amphetamines and opiates.
Catheter	In medicine, a catheter is a tube that can be inserted into a body cavity, duct, or vessel. catheters thereby allow drainage, injection of fluids, or access by surgical instruments. The process of inserting a catheter is catheterization.

Urostomy

A Urostomy is a stoma (artificial opening) for the urinary system. A Urostomy is made in cases where long-term drainage of urine through the bladder and urethra is not possible, e.g. after extensive surgery or in case of obstruction.

A `continent Urostomy` is an artificial bladder formed out of a segment of small bowel.

Urethra

In anatomy, the urethra is a tube which connects the urinary bladder to the outside of the body. In males, the urethra travels through the penis, and carries semen as well as urine. In females, the urethra is shorter and emerges above the vaginal opening.

Catheterization

In medicine a catheter is a tube that can be inserted into a body cavity, duct or vessel. Catheters thereby allow drainage, injection of fluids or access by surgical instruments. The process of inserting a catheter is catheterization.

Urinary catheterization

In Urinary catheterization, a plastic tube known as a urinary catheter is inserted into a patient`s bladder via their urethra. Catheterization allows the patient`s urine to drain freely from the bladder for collection, or to inject liquids used for treatment or diagnosis of bladder conditions. The procedure of catheterization will usually be done by a clinician, often a nurse, although self-catheterization is possible as well. class=thumbinner style="WIDTH: 182px"> class=magnify> Catheters come in several basic designs:

· A Foley catheter is retained by means of a balloon at the tip which is inflated with sterile water.

Urinary incontinence

Urinary incontinence is any involuntary leakage of urine. It is a common and distressing problem, which may have a profound impact on quality of life. urinary incontinence almost always results from an underlying treatable medical condition.

Urinary tract infection

A urinary tract infection is a bacterial infection that affects any part of the urinary tract. The main causitive agent is Escherichia coli. Although urine contains a variety of fluids, salts, and waste products, it usually does not have bacteria in it.

Urge incontinence

Urge incontinence is a form of urinary incontinence.

	Urge incontinence is involuntary loss of urine occurring for no apparent reason while suddenly feeling the need or urge to urinate. The most common cause of Urge incontinence is involuntary and inappropriate detrusor muscle contractions.
Instability	Instability in systems is generally characterized by some of the outputs or internal states growing without bounds. Not all systems that are not stable are unstable; systems can also be marginally stable or exhibit limit cycle behavior. In control theory, a system is unstable if any of the roots of its characteristic equation has real part greater than zero.
Overflow incontinence	Overflow incontinence is a form of urinary incontinence. Sometimes people find that they cannot stop their bladders from constantly dribbling, or continuing to dribble for some time after they have passed urine. It is as if their bladders were like a constantly overflowing pan, hence the general name Overflow incontinence.
Valsalva maneuver	The Valsalva maneuver or Valsalva manoeuvre is performed by forcible exhalation against a closed airway, usually done by closing one`s mouth and pinching one`s nose shut. Variations of the maneuver can be used either in medical examination as a test of cardiac function and autonomic nervous control of the heart, or to `clear` the ears and sinuses (that is, to equalize pressure between them) when ambient pressure changes, as in diving or aviation. The technique is named after Antonio Maria Valsalva, the 17th Century physician and anatomist from Bologna, whose principal scientific interest was the human ear.
Adaptation	Adaptation is the process whereby a population becomes better suited to its habitat. This process takes place over many generations, and is one of the basic phenomena of biology. The significance of an Adaptation can only be understood in relation to the total biology of the species.

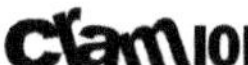

Maladaptation	A Maladaptation is an adaptation that is (or has become) more harmful than helpful. It is a term used when discussing both humans and animals in fields such as evolutionary biology, biology, psychology (where it applies to behaviors and other learned survival mechanisms), sociology, and other fields where adaptation and responsive change may occur. Like adaptation, it may be viewed as occurring over geological time, or within the lifetime of one individual or a group.
Mumps	Mumps and epidemic parotitis is a viral disease of the human species, caused by the mumps virus. Prior to the development of vaccination and the introduction of a vaccine, it was a common childhood disease worldwide, and is still a significant threat to health in the third world. Painful swelling of the salivary glands (classically the parotid gland) is the most typical presentation.
Elder abuse	Elder abuse is a general term used to describe certain types of harm to older adults. Other terms commonly used include: 'elder mistreatment', 'senior abuse', 'abuse in later life', 'abuse of older adults', 'abuse of older women', and 'abuse of older men'. One of the more commonly accepted definitions of Elder abuse is 'a single, or repeated act, or lack of appropriate action, occurring within any relationship where there is an expectation of trust which causes harm or distress to an older person.' This definition has been adopted by the World Health Organization from a definition put forward by Action on Elder abuse in the UK. The core feature of this definition is that it focuses on harms where there is 'expectation of trust' of the older person toward their abuser.
Dysfunctional families	A dysfunctional family is a family in which conflict, misbehavior and even abuse on the part of individual members of the family occur continually and regularly, leading other members to accommodate such actions. Children sometimes grow up in such families with the understanding that such an arrangement is normal. Dysfunctional families are primarily a result of co-dependent adults, and also affected by the alcoholism, substance abuse, or other addictions of parents, parents' untreated mental illnesses/defects or personality disorders, or the parents emulating their own dysfunctional parents and family experiences.
Histoplasmosis	Histoplasmosis is a disease caused by the fungus Histoplasma capsulatum. Symptoms of this infection vary greatly, but the disease primarily affects the lungs. Occasionally, other organs are affected; this is called disseminated histoplasmosis, and it can be fatal if left untreated. Histoplasmosis is common among AIDS patients because of their suppressed immune system.

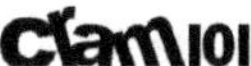

Focus groups	A focus group is a form of qualitative research in which a group of people are asked about their perceptions, opinions, beliefs and attitudes towards a product, service, concept, advertisement, idea, or packaging. Questions are asked in an interactive group setting where participants are free to talk with other group members. The first Focus groups were created at the Bureau of Applied Social Research by associate director, sociologist Robert K. Merton.
Immunization	Immunization, is the process by which an individual`s immune system becomes fortified against an agent (known as the immunogen). When an immune system is exposed to molecules that are foreign to the body (non-self), it will orchestrate an immune response, but it can also develop the ability to quickly respond to a subsequent encounter (through immunological memory). This is a function of the adaptive immune system.
Pulmonary edema	Pulmonary edema is fluid accumulation in the lungs. It leads to impaired gas exchange and may cause respiratory failure. It is due to either failure of the heart to remove fluid from the lung circulation or a direct injury to the lung parenchyma (`noncardiogenic pulmonary edema`).
Heart failure	Heart failure is a condition in which a problem with the structure or function of the heart impairs its ability to supply sufficient blood flow to meet the body`s needs. The phrase is often wrongly used to describe other cardiac-related illnesses, such as myocardial infarction (heart attack) or cardiac arrest. Common causes of Heart failure include myocardial infarction and other forms of ischemic heart disease, hypertension, valvular heart disease and cardiomyopathy.
Venous thrombosis	A venous thrombosis is a blood clot that forms within a vein. (Thrombosis is a specific medical term for a blood clot that remains in the place where it formed). Superficial venous thromboses can cause discomfort but generally do not cause serious consequences, unlike the deep venous thromboses (DVTs) that form in the deep veins of the legs or in the pelvic veins.
Hypovolemia	In physiology and medicine, Hypovolemia (also hypovolaemia) is a state of decreased blood volume ; more specifically, decrease in volume of blood plasma. It is thus the intravascular component of volume contraction (or loss of blood volume due to things such as hemorrhaging or dehydration), but, as it also is the most essential one, Hypovolemia and volume contraction are sometimes used synonymously. It differs from dehydration, which is defined as excessive loss of body water.

Acid-base imbalance	Acid-base imbalance is an abnormality of the human body's normal balance of acids and bases that causes the plasma pH to deviate out of the normal range (7.35 to 7.45). It can exist in varying levels of severity, some life-threatening. An excess of acid is called acidosis (pH less than 7.35) and an excess in bases is called alkalosis (pH greater than 7.45).
Acidosis	Acidosis is an increased acidity (i.e. an increased hydrogen ion concentration). If not further qualified, it usually refers to acidity of the blood plasma. Acidosis is said to occur when arterial pH falls below 7.35, while its counterpart (alkalosis) occurs at a pH over 7.45. Arterial blood gas analysis and other tests are required to separate the main causes.
Alkalosis	Alkalosis refers to a condition reducing hydrogen ion concentration of arterial blood plasma (alkalemia). Generally Alkalosis is said to occur when pH of the blood exceeds 7.45. The opposite condition is acidosis. More specifically, Alkalosis can refer to: · Respiratory Alkalosis · Metabolic Alkalosis The main cause of respiratory Alkalosis is hyperventilation, resulting in a loss of carbon dioxide. Compensatory mechanisms for this would include increased dissociation of the carbonic acid buffering intermediate into hydrogen ions, and the related excretion of bicarbonate, both of which would lower blood pH.
Atelectasis	Atelectasis is defined as the lack of gas exchange within alveoli, due to alveolar collapse or fluid consolidation. It may affect part or all of one lung. It is a condition where the alveoli are deflated, as distinct from pulmonary consolidation.

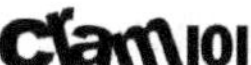

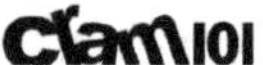

	It is a very common finding in chest x-rays and other radiological studies. It may be caused by normal exhalation or by several medical conditions. Although frequently described as a collapse of lung tissue, atelectasis is not synonymous with a pneumothorax, which is a more specific condition that features atelectasis. Acute atelectasis may occur as a post-operative complication or as a result of surfactant deficiency. In premature neonates, this leads to infant respiratory distress syndrome.
Septic	Septic is a word derived from the Greek ΣÎ®ψις, meaning `putrefaction`. Septic may refer to: · a Septic infection, cf. sepsis · Septic tank or Septic system a simple, small scale, method of sewage disposal · Cockney rhyming slang for American, coming from Septic tank = Yank · Septic equation, a polynomial of degree seven (also called heptic, septemic or septimic)
Septic shock	Septic shock is a serious medical condition caused by decreased tissue perfusion and oxygen delivery as a result of infection and sepsis, though the microbe may be systemic or localized to a particular site. It can cause multiple organ dysfunction syndrome (formerly known as multiple organ failure) and death. Its most common victims are children, immunocompromised individuals, and the elderly, as their immune systems cannot deal with the infection as effectively as those of healthy adults.
Pneumothorax	In medicine (pulmonology), a pneumothorax is a potential medical emergency wherein air or gas is present in the pleural cavity. A pneumothorax can occur spontaneously. It can also occur as the result of disease or injury to the lung, or due to a puncture to the chest wall.
Asthma	Asthma is characterized by a predisposition to chronic inflammation of the lungs in which the airways (bronchi) are reversibly narrowed. Asthma affects 7% of the population of the United States 6.5% of British people and a total of 300 million worldwide. During Asthma attacks (exacerbations of Asthma), the smooth muscle cells in the bronchi constrict, the airways become inflamed and swollen, and breathing becomes difficult.

Chapter 3. PART III: Chapter 5 - Chapter 6

Insulin	Insulin is a hormone that has profound effects on metabolism. insulin causes cells in the liver, muscle, and fat tissue to take up glucose from the blood, storing it as glycogen in the liver and muscle, and stopping use of fat as an energy source. When insulin is absent (or low), glucose is not taken up by body cells, and the body begins to use fat as an energy source, for example, by transfer of lipids from adipose tissue to the liver for mobilization as an energy source.
Diabetes mellitus	Diabetes mellitus --often referred to simply as diabetes--is a condition in which the body either does not produce enough, insulin, a hormone produced in the pancreas. Insulin enables cells to absorb glucose in order to turn it into energy. In diabetes, the body either fails to properly respond to its own insulin, does not make enough insulin, or both.
Mellitus	Mellitus was the first Bishop of London, the third Archbishop of Canterbury, and a member of the Gregorian mission sent to England to convert the Anglo-Saxons. He arrived in 601 AD with a group of clergymen sent to augment the mission, and was consecrated as Bishop of London in 604. Mellitus was the recipient of a famous letter from Pope Gregory I known as the Epistola ad Mellitum, preserved in a later work by the medieval chronicler Bede, which suggested the conversion of the Anglo-Saxons be undertaken gradually and integrate pagan rituals and customs. In 610, Mellitus returned to Italy to attend a council of bishops, and returned to England bearing papal letters to some of the missionaries.
Coma	In medicine, a Coma is a profound state of unconsciousness. A person in a Coma cannot be awakened, fails to respond normally to pain, light or sound, does not have sleep-wake cycles, and does not take voluntary actions. A person in a state of Coma can be described as Comatose.
Cachexia	Cachexia is loss of weight, muscle atrophy, fatigue, weakness and significant loss of appetite in someone who is not actively trying to lose weight. The formal definition of Cachexia is the loss of body mass that cannot be reversed nutritionally; even if you supplement the patient calorically, lean body mass will be lost, indicating there is a fundamental pathology in place. Cachexia is seen in patients with cancer, AIDS, COPD , CHF (congestive heart failure) and Familial Amyloid Polyneuropathy.
Hypoalbuminemia	Hypoalbuminemia is a medical condition where levels of albumin in blood serum are abnormally low. It is a specific form of hypoproteinemia.
	Albumin is a major protein in the human body, making up about 60% of total human plasma protein by mass.

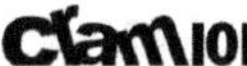

Hypokalemia	Hypokalemia , or hypokalaemia , refers to the condition in which the concentration of potassium (K^+) in the blood is low. The prefix hypo- means low (contrast with hyper-, meaning high). Kal refers to kalium, the Neo-Latin for potassium, and -emia means `in the blood.` Normal serum potassium levels are between 3.5 to 5.0 mEq/L; at least 95% of the body`s potassium is found inside cells, with the remainder in the blood.
Parenteral	Parenteral is a route of administration that involves piercing the skin or mucous membrane. Parenteral nutrition refers to providing nutrition via the veins. From Greek para = `beside` and enteron = `intestine`, because it bypasses the intestines.
Parenteral nutrition	Parenteral nutrition is feeding a person intravenously, bypassing the usual process of eating and digestion. The person receives nutritional formulas containing salts, glucose, amino acids, lipids and added vitamins. It is called total Parenteral nutrition when no food is given by other routes.
Potassium	Potassium is the chemical element with the symbol K , atomic number 19, and atomic mass 39.0983. potassium was first isolated from potash. Elemental potassium is a soft silvery-white metallic alkali metal that oxidizes rapidly in air and is very reactive with water, generating sufficient heat to ignite the evolved hydrogen. potassium in nature occurs only as ionic salt.
Hyperkalemia	Hyperkalemia is an elevated blood level of the electrolyte potassium. Extreme hyperkalemia is a medical emergency due to the risk of potentially fatal abnormal heart rhythms (arrhythmia). Symptoms are fairly nonspecific and generally include malaise, palpitations and muscle weakness; mild hyperventilation may indicate a compensatory response to metabolic acidosis, which is one of the possible causes of hyperkalemia.
Hypernatremia	Hypernatremia or hypernatraemia is an electrolyte disturbance that is defined by an elevated sodium level in the blood. hypernatremia is generally not caused by an excess of sodium, but rather by a relative deficit of free water in the body. For this reason, hypernatremia is often synonymous with the less precise term, dehydration.

Hyponatremia	Hyponatremia is an electrolyte disturbance (a disturbance of the salts in the blood) in which the sodium concentration in the plasma is lower than normal . Severe or rapidly progressing hyponatremia can result in swelling of the brain (cerebral edema), and the symptoms of hyponatremia are mainly neurological. hyponatremia is most often a complication of other medical illnesses in which either fluids rich in sodium are lost (for example because of diarrhea or vomiting), or excess water accumulates in the body at a higher rate than it can be excreted (for example in polydipsia or syndrome of inappropriate antidiuretic hormone, SIADH).
Sodium	Sodium is a metallic element with a symbol Na and atomic number 11. It is a soft, silvery-white, highly reactive metal and is a member of the alkali metals within `group 1` (formerly known as `group IA`). It has only one stable isotope, ^{23}Na. Elemental sodium was first isolated by Sir Humphry Davy in 1806 by passing an electric current through molten sodium hydroxide.
Calcium	Calcium is the chemical element with the symbol Ca and atomic number 20. It has an atomic mass of 40.078 amu. calcium is a soft gray alkaline earth metal, and is the fifth most abundant element by mass in the Earth's crust. calcium is also the fifth most abundant dissolved ion in seawater by both molarity and mass, after sodium, chloride, magnesium, and sulfate.
Hyperphosphatemia	Hyperphosphatemia is an electrolyte disturbance in which there is an abnormally elevated level of phosphate in the blood. Often, calcium levels are lowered (hypocalcemia) due to precipitation of phosphate with the calcium in tissues. Hypoparathyroidism: In this situation, there are low levels of Parathyroid hormone (PTH).
Hypocalcemia	In medicine, hypocalcemia is the presence of low serum calcium levels in the blood, usually taken as less than 2.1 mmol/L or 9 mg/dl or an ionized calcium level mm of less than 1.1 mmol/L (4.5 mg/dL). It is a type of electrolyte disturbance. In the blood, about half of all calcium is bound to proteins such as serum albumin, but it is the unbound, or ionized, calcium that the body regulates.
Hypomagnesemia	Hypomagnesemia is an electrolyte disturbance in which there is an abnormally low level of magnesium in the blood. Usually a serum level less than 0.7 mmol/L is used as reference. hypomagnesemia is not equal to magnesium deficiency.

Hypophosphatemia	Hypophosphatemia is an electrolyte disturbance in which there is an abnormally low level of phosphate in the blood. The condition has many causes, but is most commonly seen when malnourished patients (especially chronic alcoholics) are given large amounts of carbohydrates, which creates a high phosphorus demand by cells, removing phosphate from the blood (refeeding syndrome). Because a decrease in phosphate in the blood is sometimes associated with an increase in phosphate in the urine, the terms Hypophosphatemia and `phosphaturia` are occasionally used interchangeably; however, this is improper since there exist many causes of Hypophosphatemia besides overexcretion and phosphaturia, and in fact the most common causes of Hypophosphatemia are not associated with phosphaturia. · Refeeding syndrome This causes a demand for phosphate in cells due to the action of phosphofructokinase, an enzyme which attaches phosphate to glucose to begin metabolism of this.
Phosphate	A phosphate, an inorganic chemical, is a salt of phosphoric acid. In organic chemistry, a phosphate, or organophosphate, is an ester of phosphoric acid. Organic phosphates are important in biochemistry and biogeochemistry or ecology.
Hyperchloremia	Hyperchloremia is an electrolyte disturbance in which there is an abnormally elevated level of the chloride ion in the blood. The normal serum range for chloride is 97 to 107 mEq/L. Hyperchloremia is defined as a chloride concentration exceeding this level. Hyperchloremia can affect oxygen transport.
Hypermagnesemia	Hypermagnesemia is an electrolyte disturbance in which there is an abnormally elevated level of magnesium in the blood. Usually this results in excess of magnesium in the body. hypermagnesemia occurs rarely because the kidney is very effective in excreting excess magnesium.

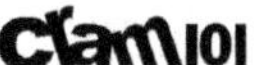

Hypochloremia	Hypochloremia is an electrolyte disturbance whereby there is an abnormally depleted level of the chloride ion in the blood. It rarely occurs in the absence of other abnormalities. It can be associated with hypoventilation.
Magnesium	Magnesium is a chemical element with the symbol Mg, atomic number 12 and common oxidation number +2. It is an alkaline earth metal and the eighth most abundant element in the Earth`s crust by mass, although ninth in the Universe as a whole. This preponderance of magnesium is related to the fact that it is easily built up in supernova stars from a sequential addition of three helium nuclei to carbon . magnesium constitutes about 2% of the Earth`s crust by mass, which makes it the eighth most abundant element in the crust.
Metabolic acidosis	In medicine, metabolic acidosis is a process which if unchecked leads to acidemia, i.e. blood pH is low (less than 7.35) due to increased production of H^+ by the body or the inability of the body to form bicarbonate (HCO_3^-) in the kidney. Its causes are diverse, and its consequences can be serious, including coma and death. Together with respiratory acidosis, it is one of the two general causes of acidemia.
Respiratory acidosis	Respiratory acidosis is a medical condition in which decreased respiration (hypoventilation) causes increased blood carbon dioxide and decreased pH (a condition generally called acidosis). Carbon dioxide is produced constantly as the body burns energy, and this CO_2 will accumulate rapidly if the lungs do not adequately dispel it through alveolar ventilation. Alveolar hypoventilation thus leads to an increased $PaCO_2$ (called hypercapnia).
Metabolic alkalosis	Metabolic alkalosis is a metabolic condition in which the pH of the blood is elevated beyond the normal range (7.35-7.45). This is usually the result of decreased hydrogen ion concentration, leading to increased bicarbonate, or alternatively a direct result of increased bicarbonate concentrations. There are five main causes of metabolic alkalosis.

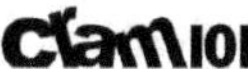

Respiratory alkalosis	Respiratory alkalosis is a medical condition in which increased respiration (hyperventilation) elevates the blood pH (a condition generally called alkalosis). It is one of four basic categories of disruption of acid-base homeostasis. There are two types of respiratory alkalosis: chronic and acute. · Acute respiratory alkalosis occurs rapidly.
Thrombocytopenia	Thrombocytopenia is the presence of relatively few platelets in blood. Generally speaking, in human beings a normal platelet count ranges from 150,000 to 450,000 platelets per microliter of blood. These limits, however, are determined by the 2.5th lower and upper percentile, and a deviation does not necessarily imply any form of disease.
Opportunistic infection	An opportunistic infection is an infection caused by pathogens (bacterial, viral, fungal or protozoan) that usually do not cause disease in a healthy host, i.e. one with a healthy immune system. A compromised immune system, however, presents an `opportunity` for the pathogen to infect.
Anticoagulant	An Anticoagulant is a substance that prevents coagulation; that is, it stops blood from clotting. A group of pharmaceuticals called Anticoagulants can be used in vivo as a medication for thrombotic disorders. Some chemical compounds are used in medical equipment, such as test tubes, blood transfusion bags, and renal dialysis equipment.
Chest	The Chest is a part of the anatomy of humans and various other animals sometimes referred to as the thorax. In hominids, the Chest is the region of the body between the neck and the abdomen, along with its internal organs and other contents. It is mostly protected and supported by the ribcage, spine, and shoulder girdle. Contents of the Chest include the following: · organs · heart

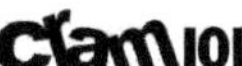

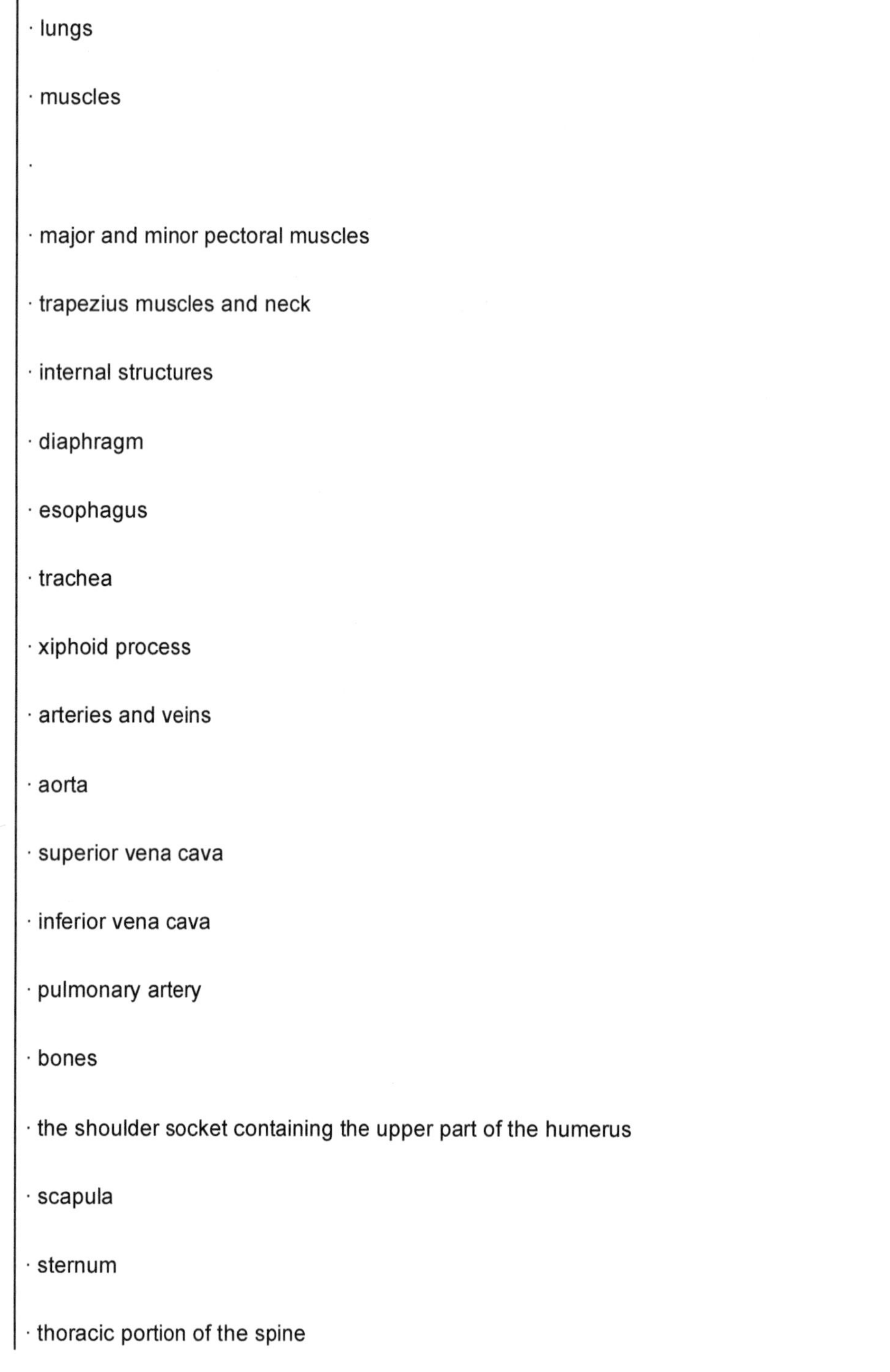

· lungs

· muscles

·

· major and minor pectoral muscles

· trapezius muscles and neck

· internal structures

· diaphragm

· esophagus

· trachea

· xiphoid process

· arteries and veins

· aorta

· superior vena cava

· inferior vena cava

· pulmonary artery

· bones

· the shoulder socket containing the upper part of the humerus

· scapula

· sternum

· thoracic portion of the spine

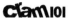

· collarbone

· ribcage

· Floating ribs

· external structures

· nipples

· mammary glands

· The V of the Chest is the area exposed by open-necked shirts.

· thoracic abdomen
In humans, the portion of the Chest protected by the ribcage is also called the thorax.

Oliguria

Oliguria is the decreased production of urine. The decreased production of urine may be a sign of dehydration, renal failure, hypovolemic shock or urinary obstruction/urinary retention.

It can be contrasted with anuria, which represents a more complete suppression of urination.

Pyelonephritis

Pyelonephritis is an ascending urinary tract infection that has reached the pyelum (pelvis) of the kidney . If the infection is severe, the term `urosepsis` is used interchangeably . It requires antibiotics as therapy, and treatment of any underlying causes to prevent recurrence.

Seizure

An epileptic seizure is a transient symptom of excessive or synchronous neuronal activity in the brain. It can manifest as an alteration in mental state, tonic or clonic movements, convulsions, and various other psychic symptoms (such as déjà vu or jamais vu). The medical syndrome of recurrent, unprovoked seizures is termed epilepsy, but seizures can occur in people who do not have epilepsy.

Convulsions

A convulsion is a medical condition where body muscles contract and relax rapidly and repeatedly, resulting in an uncontrolled shaking of the body. Because a convulsion is often a symptom of an epileptical seizure, the term convulsion is sometimes used as a synonym for seizure. However, not all epileptic seizures lead to Convulsions, and not all Convulsions are caused by epileptic seizures.

Status epilepticus	Status epilepticus is a life-threatening condition in which the brain is in a state of persistent seizure. Definitions vary, but traditionally it is defined as one continuous unremitting seizure lasting longer than 30 minutes , or recurrent seizures without regaining consciousness between seizures for greater than 30 minutes (or shorter with medical intervention). There is some evidence that 5 minutes is sufficient to damage neurons and that seizures are unlikely to self-terminate by that time.
Glaucoma	Glaucoma is a disease that affects the optic nerve and involves loss of retinal ganglion cells in a characteristic pattern. There are many different sub-types of Glaucoma but they can all be considered as a type of optic neuropathy. Raised intraocular pressure is a significant risk factor for developing Glaucoma (above 22 mmHg or 2.9 kPa).
Intraocular pressure	Intraocular pressure is the fluid pressure of the aqueous humor inside the eye. In ophthalmology, tonometry is the measurement eye care professionals use to determine the fluid pressure inside the eye. IOP is an important aspect in the evaluation of patients with glaucoma. Most tonometers are calibrated to measure pressure in millimeters of mercury (mmHg).
Malignant	Malignancy is the tendency of a medical condition, especially tumors to become progressively worse and to potentially result in death. It is characterized by the properties of anaplasia, invasiveness, and metastasis. Malignant is a corresponding adjectival medical term used to describe a severe and progressively worsening disease.
Neuroleptic malignant syndrome	Neuroleptic malignant syndrome is a life- threatening neurological disorder most often caused by an adverse reaction to neuroleptic or antipsychotic drugs. It generally presents with muscle rigidity, fever, autonomic instability and cognitive changes such as delirium, and is associated with elevated creatine phosphokinase (CPK). Incidence of the disease has declined since its discovery (due to changes in prescription habits), but it is still a potential danger to patients being treated with antipsychotics.
Dantrolene	Dantrolene sodium is a muscle relaxant that acts by abolishing excitation-contraction coupling in muscle cells, probably by action on the ryanodine receptor. It is the only specific and effective treatment for malignant hyperthermia, a rare, life-threatening disorder triggered by general anesthesia. It is also used in the management of neuroleptic malignant syndrome, muscle spasticity (e.g. after strokes, in paraplegia, cerebral palsy, or patients with multiple sclerosis), ecstasy intoxication, serotonin syndrome, and 2,4-dinitrophenol poisoning.

Extrapyramidal symptoms

The extrapyramidal system can be affected in a number of ways, which are revealed in a range of Extrapyramidal symptoms such as akinesia (inability to initiate movement) and akathisia (inability to remain motionless).

Extrapyramidal symptoms are the various movement disorders such as tardive dyskinesia suffered as a result of taking dopamine antagonists, usually antipsychotic (neuroleptic) drugs, which are often used to control psychosis.

The Simpson-Angus Scale (SAS) and the Barnes Akathisia Rating Scale (BARS) are used to measure Extrapyramidal symptoms.

Dysphagia

Dysphagia is the medical term for the symptom of difficulty in swallowing. Although classified under 'symptoms and signs' in ICD-10, the term is sometimes used as a condition in its own right. Sufferers are sometimes unaware of their Dysphagia.

Benzodiazepine

A Benzodiazepine is a psychoactive drug whose core chemical structure is the fusion of a benzene ring and a diazepine ring. The first Benzodiazepine, chlordiazepoxide , was discovered accidentally by Leo Sternbach in 1955, and made available in 1960 by Hoffmann-La Roche, which has also marketed diazepam (Valium) since 1963.

Benzodiazepines enhance the effect of the neurotransmitter gamma-aminobutyric acid, which results in sedative, hypnotic (sleep-inducing), anxiolytic (anti-anxiety), anticonvulsant, muscle relaxant and amnesic action.

Bowel obstruction

Bowel obstruction (or intestinal obstruction) is a mechanical or functional obstruction of the intestines, preventing the normal transit of the products of digestion. It can occur at any level distal to the duodenum of the small intestine and is a medical emergency. Although many cases are not treated surgically, it is a surgical problem.

class=thumbinner style="WIDTH: 182px"> class=magnify> class=thumbinner style="WIDTH: 182px"> class=magnify>
Causes of small Bowel obstruction include:

· Adhesions from previous abdominal surgery

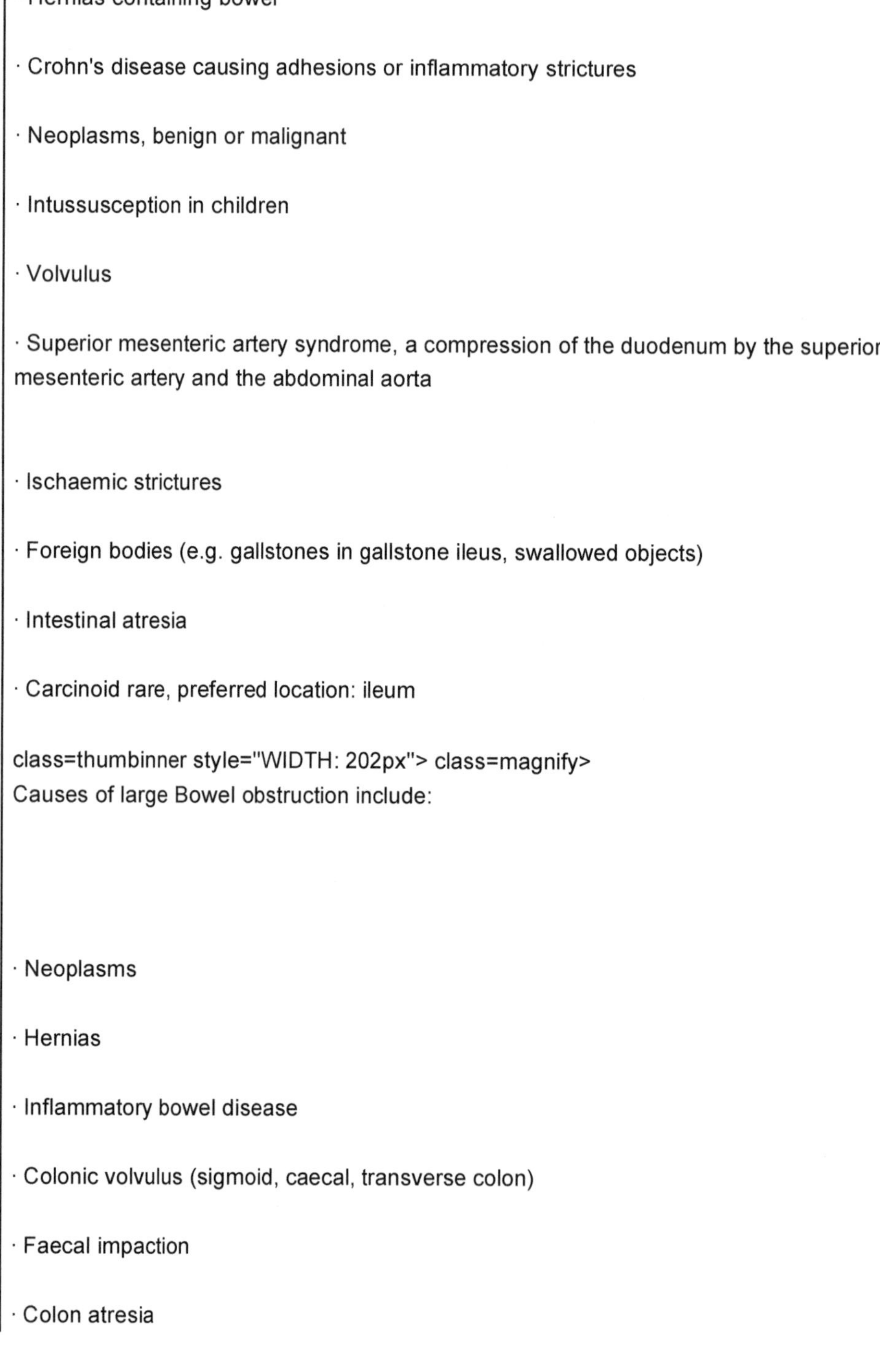

· Hernias containing bowel

· Crohn's disease causing adhesions or inflammatory strictures

· Neoplasms, benign or malignant

· Intussusception in children

· Volvulus

· Superior mesenteric artery syndrome, a compression of the duodenum by the superior mesenteric artery and the abdominal aorta

· Ischaemic strictures

· Foreign bodies (e.g. gallstones in gallstone ileus, swallowed objects)

· Intestinal atresia

· Carcinoid rare, preferred location: ileum

class=thumbinner style="WIDTH: 202px"> class=magnify>
Causes of large Bowel obstruction include:

· Neoplasms

· Hernias

· Inflammatory bowel disease

· Colonic volvulus (sigmoid, caecal, transverse colon)

· Faecal impaction

· Colon atresia

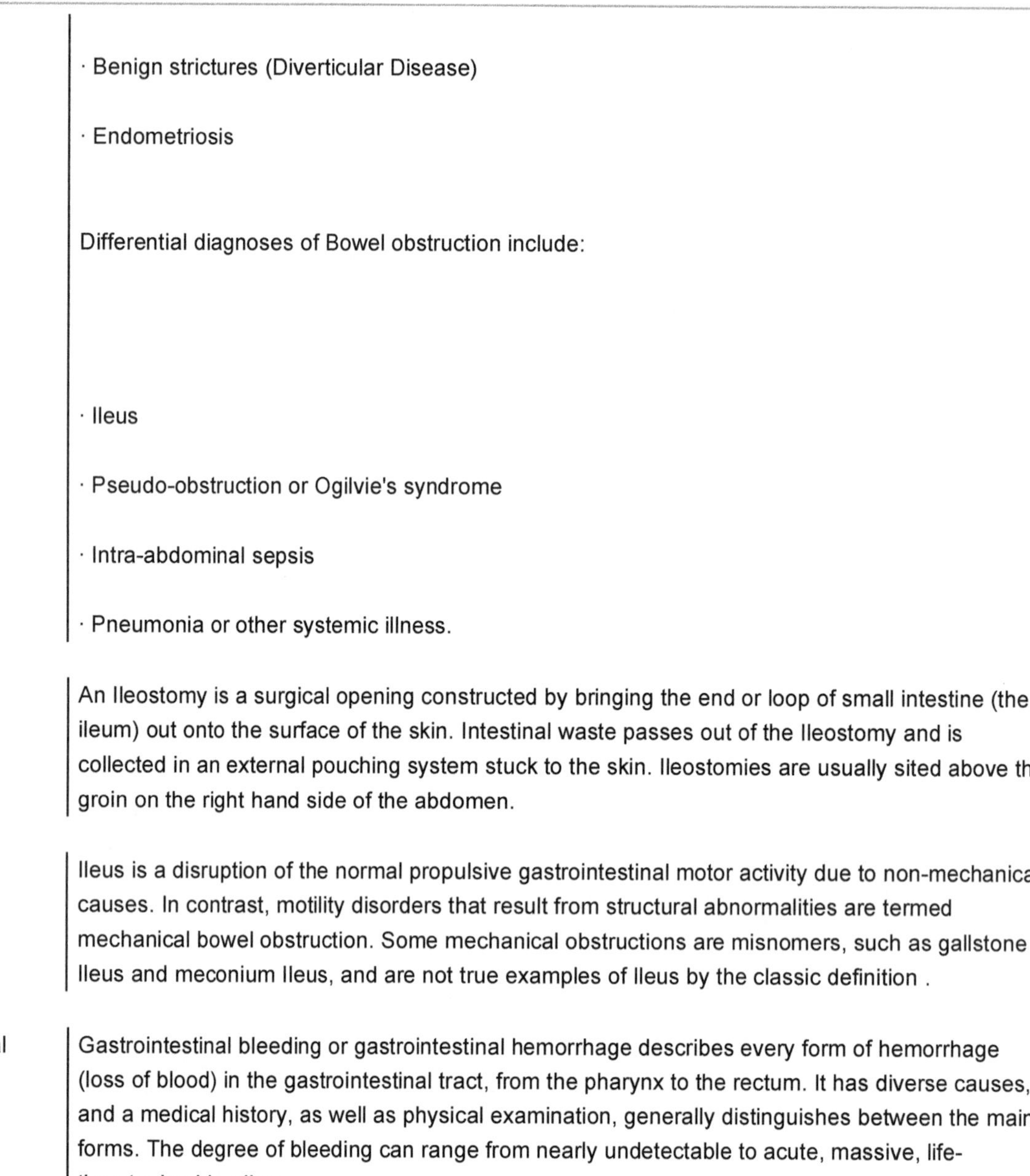

	· Benign strictures (Diverticular Disease) · Endometriosis Differential diagnoses of Bowel obstruction include: · Ileus · Pseudo-obstruction or Ogilvie's syndrome · Intra-abdominal sepsis · Pneumonia or other systemic illness.
Ileostomy	An Ileostomy is a surgical opening constructed by bringing the end or loop of small intestine (the ileum) out onto the surface of the skin. Intestinal waste passes out of the Ileostomy and is collected in an external pouching system stuck to the skin. Ileostomies are usually sited above the groin on the right hand side of the abdomen.
Ileus	Ileus is a disruption of the normal propulsive gastrointestinal motor activity due to non-mechanical causes. In contrast, motility disorders that result from structural abnormalities are termed mechanical bowel obstruction. Some mechanical obstructions are misnomers, such as gallstone Ileus and meconium Ileus, and are not true examples of Ileus by the classic definition .
Gastrointestinal bleeding	Gastrointestinal bleeding or gastrointestinal hemorrhage describes every form of hemorrhage (loss of blood) in the gastrointestinal tract, from the pharynx to the rectum. It has diverse causes, and a medical history, as well as physical examination, generally distinguishes between the main forms. The degree of bleeding can range from nearly undetectable to acute, massive, life-threatening bleeding.

Gastric	In most mammals, the stomach is a hollow, muscular organ of the gastrointestinal tract (digestive system), between the esophagus and the small intestine. It is involved in the second phase of digestion, following mastication (chewing). The word stomach is derived from the Latin stomachus which is derived from the Greek word stomachos which is derived from the word gastro- and gastric are both derived from the Greek word gaster (γαστÎ®ρ).
Bilirubin	Bilirubin is the yellow breakdown product of normal heme catabolism. Heme is found in hemoglobin, a principal component of red blood cells. Bilirubin is excreted in bile and urine, and elevated levels may indicate certain diseases.
Encephalopathy	Encephalopathy /É›nËŒsÉ›fÉ™ËˆlÉ’pÉ™θi/ literally means disorder or disease of the brain. In modern usage, Encephalopathy does not refer to a single disease, but rather to a syndrome of global brain dysfunction; this syndrome can be caused by many different illnesses. In some contexts it refers to permanent (or degenerative) brain injury, and in others it is reversible.
Hyperbilirubinemia	Jaundice, also known as icterus (attributive adjective: icteric), is a yellowish discoloration of the skin, the conjunctival membranes over the sclerae (whites of the eyes), and other mucous membranes caused by hyperbilirubinemia. This hyperbilirubinemia subsequently causes increased levels of bilirubin in the extracellular fluids. Typically, the concentration of bilirubin in the plasma must exceed 1.5 mg/dL, three times the usual value of approximately 0.5 mg/dL, for the coloration to be easily visible.
Jaundice	Jaundice, also known as icterus (attributive adjective: icteric), is a yellowish discoloration of the skin, the conjunctival membranes over the sclerae (whites of the eyes), and other mucous membranes caused by hyperbilirubinemia (increased levels of bilirubin in the blood). This hyperbilirubinemia subsequently causes increased levels of bilirubin in the extracellular fluids. Typically, the concentration of bilirubin in the plasma must exceed 1.5 mg/dL, three times the usual value of approximately 0.5 mg/dL, for the coloration to be easily visible.
Systemic	Systemic refers to something that is spread throughout, system-wide, affecting a group or system such as a body, economy, market or society as a whole. It should not be confused with \`systematic\`, which means methodical. Systemic may also refer to: In medicine, Systemic means affecting the whole body, or at least multiple organ systems.

Musculoskeletal

A musculoskeletal system (also known as the locomotor system) is an organ system that gives animals (including humans) the ability to move using the muscular and skeletal systems. The musculoskeletal system provides form, stability, and movement to the body.

It is made up of the body`s bones (the skeleton), muscles, cartilage, tendons, ligaments, joints, and other connective tissue (the tissue that supports and binds tissues and organs together).

Shoulder

In human anatomy, the Shoulder joint comprises the part of the body where the humerus attaches to the scapula. The Shoulder is the group of structures in the region of the joint.

It is made up of three bones: the clavicle , the scapula (Shoulder blade), and the humerus (upper arm bone) as well as associated muscles, ligaments and tendons.

Dysplasia

Dysplasia is a term used in pathology to refer to an abnormality in maturation of cells within a tissue. This generally consists of an expansion of immature cells, with a corresponding decrease in the number and location of mature cells. Dysplasia is often indicative of an early neoplastic process.

Placenta

The Placenta is an organ that connects the developing fetus to the uterine wall to allow nutrient uptake, waste elimination and gas exchange via the mother`s blood supply. Placentas are a defining characteristic of eutherian or `Placental` mammals, but are also found in some snakes and lizards with varying levels of development up to mammalian levels. The word Placenta comes from the Latin for cake, from Greek plakóenta/plakoúnta, accusative of plakóeis/plakoús - πλακÏŒεις, πλακοÏ ς, `flat, slab-like`, in reference to its round, flat appearance in humans.

Placenta previa

Placenta praevia (placenta previa AE) is an obstetric complication in which the placenta is attached to the uterine wall close to or covering the cervix. It can sometimes occur in the later part of the first trimester, but usually during the second or third. It is a leading cause of antepartum haemorrhage (vaginal bleeding).

Magnesium sulfate

Magnesium sulfate is a chemical compound containing magnesium, sulfur and oxygen, with the formula $MgSO_4$. In its hydrated form the pH is 6.0 (5.5 to 6.5). It is often encountered as the heptahydrate, $MgSO_4$Â·$7H_2O$, commonly called Epsom salt.

Preterm

In humans, preterm birth refers to the birth of a baby of less than 37 weeks gestational age. Premature birth, commonly used as a synonym f birth, refers to the birth of a premature infant. The child may commonly be referred to throughout their life as being born a `preemie` or `preemie baby`.

Proteinuria	Proteinuria (/prÉ™ÊŠtiË ˈn(j)ÊŠÉ™riÉ™/, from protein and urine) means the presence of an excess of serum proteins in the urine. The protein in the urine often causes the urine to become foamy, although foamy urine may also be caused by bilirubin in the urine (bilirubinuria), retrograde ejaculation, pneumaturia (air bubbles in the urine) due to a fistula, or drugs such as pyridium. There are three main mechanisms to cause Proteinuria: 1. Due to disease in glomerulus 2. Because of increased quantity of proteins in serum (overflow Proteinuria) 3. Due to low reabsorbtion at proximal tubule (fanconi) Proteinuria is often diagnosed by a simple dipstick test although it is possible for the test to give a false negative even with nephrotic range Proteinuria if the urine is dilute.
Tachycardia	Tachycardia comes from the Greek words tachys and kardia (of the heart). tachycardia typically refers to a heart rate that exceeds the normal range for a resting heartrate (heartrate in an inactive or sleeping individual). In humans, the upper threshold of a normal heart rate is usually based upon age, sometimes it can be very dangerous depending on how hard the heart is working and the activity: · 1-2 days: >159 beats per minute (bpm) · 3-6 days: >166 bpm · 1-3 weeks: >182 bpm · 1-2 months: >179 bpm · 3-5 months: >186 bpm · 6-11 months: >169 bpm

· 1-2 years: >151 bpm

· 3-4 years: >137 bpm

· 5-7 years: >133 bpm

· 8-11 years: >130 bpm

· 12-15 years: >119 bpm

· >15 years - adult: >100 bpm

When the heart beats rapidly, the heart pumps less efficiently and provides less blood flow to the rest of the body, including the heart itself. The increased heart rate also leads to increased work and oxygen demand for the heart (myocardium), which can cause a heart attack (myocardial infarction) if it persists.

Uterus

The uterus is a major female hormone-responsive reproductive sex organ of most mammals, including humans. It is within the uterus that the fetus develops during gestation. The term uterus is used consistently within the medical and related professions; the Germanic term, womb is more common in everyday usage.

Postpartum hemorrhage

Hemorrhage after delivery, or Postpartum hemorrhage, is the loss of greater than 500 ml of blood following vaginal delivery, or 1000 ml of blood following cesarean section. It is the most common cause of perinatal maternal death in the developed world and is a major cause of maternal morbidity worldwide.

Anticoagulant

An Anticoagulant is a substance that prevents coagulation; that is, it stops blood from clotting. A group of pharmaceuticals called Anticoagulants can be used in vivo as a medication for thrombotic disorders. Some chemical compounds are used in medical equipment, such as test tubes, blood transfusion bags, and renal dialysis equipment.

Cornea

The Cornea is the transparent front part of the eye that covers the iris, pupil, and anterior chamber. Together with the lens, the Cornea refracts light, accounting for approximately two-thirds of the eye's total optical power. In humans, the refractive power of the Cornea is approximately 43 dioptres.

Antineoplastic

Antineoplastics are drugs that inhibit and combat the development of neoplasms.

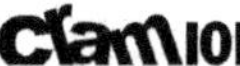

	In the Anatomical Therapeutic Chemical Classification System, they are classified under L01. The adverse health effects associated with Antineoplastic agents (cancer chemotherapy drugs, cytotoxic drugs) in cancer patients and some non-cancer patients treated with these drugs are well-documented. The very nature of antineoplastic agents makes them harmful to healthy constantly dividing cells and tissues, as well as the cancerous cells. For cancer patients with a life-threatening disease, there is a great benefit to treatment with these agents.
Extravasation	Extravasation is the leakage of a fluid out of its container. In the case of inflammation, it refers to the movement of white blood cells from the capillaries to the tissues surrounding them (diapedesis). In the case of malignant cancer metastasis it refers to cancer cells exiting the capillaries and entering organs.
Anticonvulsant	The anticonvulsants are a diverse group of pharmaceuticals used in the treatment of epileptic seizures. anticonvulsants are also increasingly being used in the treatment of bipolar disorder, since many seem to act as mood stabilizers. The goal of an anticonvulsant is to suppress the rapid and excessive firing of neurons that start a seizure. The goal of an anticonvulsant is to suppress the rapid and excessive firing of neurons that start a seizure.
Antiarrhythmic	Antiarrhythmic agents are a group of pharmaceuticals that are used to suppress fast rhythms of the heart (cardiac arrhythmias), such as atrial fibrillation, atrial flutter, ventricular tachycardia, and ventricular fibrillation. While the use of Antiarrhythmic agents to suppress atrial arrhythmias (atrial fibrillation and atrial flutter) is still in practice, it is unclear whether suppression of atrial arrhythmias will prolong life.
Antipsychotic	An Antipsychotic is a psychiatric medication primarily used to manage psychosis (e.g. delusions or hallucinations), particularly in schizophrenia and bipolar disorder. A first generation of Antipsychotics, known as typical Antipsychotics, was discovered in the 1950s. Most of the drugs in the second generation, known as atypical Antipsychotics, have been developed more recently, although the first atypical Antipsychotic, clozapine, was discovered in the 1950s and introduced clinically in the 1970s.

Antihypertensive	The antihypertensives are a class of drugs that are used to treat hypertension . Evidence suggests that reduction of the blood pressure by 5 mmHg can decrease the risk of stroke by 34%, of ischaemic heart disease by 21%, and reduce the likelihood of dementia, heart failure, and mortality from cardiovascular disease. There are many classes of antihypertensives, which lower blood pressure by different means; among the most important and most widely used are the thiazide diuretics, the ACE inhibitors, the calcium channel blockers, the beta blockers, and the angiotensin II receptor antagonists or ARBs.
Calcium channel	A Calcium channel is an ion channel which displays selective permeabiltiy to calcium ions. It is sometimes synonymous as voltage-dependent calcium channel, although there are also ligand-gated calcium channels.
Calcium channel blocker	Calcium channel blockers are a class of drugs and natural substances that disrupt the movement of calcium (Ca^{2+}) through calcium channels. Calcium channel blockers have effects on many excitable cells of the body, such as cardiac muscle, i.e. heart, smooth muscles of blood vessels, or neurons. Drugs used to target neurons are used as antiepileptics and are not covered in this article.
Enzyme	Enzymes are proteins that catalyze (i.e., increase the rates of) chemical reactions. In enzymatic reactions, the molecules at the beginning of the process are called substrates, and the Enzyme converts them into different molecules, called the products. Almost all processes in a biological cell need Enzymes to occur at significant rates.

Lightning Source UK Ltd.
Milton Keynes UK
UKHW052027081121
393634UK00002B/25

9 781618 124579